DRUG SYNERGISM and DOSE-EFFECT DATA ANALYSIS

DRUG
SYNERGISM and
DOSE-EFFECT
DATA ANALYSIS

Ronald J. Tallarida

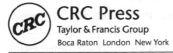

CRC Press
Taylor & Francis Group
Boca Raton London New York

CRC Press is an imprint of the
Taylor & Francis Group, an **informa** business

A CHAPMAN & HALL BOOK

CRC Press
Taylor & Francis Group
6000 Broken Sound Parkway NW, Suite 300
Boca Raton, FL 33487-2742

First issued in paperback 2019

© 2000 by Taylor & Francis Group, LLC
CRC Press is an imprint of Taylor & Francis Group, an Informa business

No claim to original U.S. Government works

ISBN-13: 978-1-58488-045-5 (hbk)
ISBN-13: 978-0-367-39834-7 (pbk)

Library of Congress Cataloging-in-Publication Data

Tallarida, Ronald J.
    Drug synergism and dose-effect analysis / Ronald J. Tallarida
        p.   cm.
    Includes bibliographical references and index.
    ISBN 1-58488-045-7 (alk. paper)
    1. Drug synergism. 2. Drug synergism—Mathematics. 3. Probits. 4.
Drugs—Dose-response relationship—Mathematics. I. Title.
    [DNLM: 1. Drug Synergism. 2. Data Interpretation, Statistical. 3. Dose-Response
Relationship, Drug. 4. Drug Therapy, Combination. 5. Regression Analysis. QV 38
T147da 2000]
    Rm302.3 .T35 2000
    615'.7—dc21   00-031433
                                                                                          CIP

Visit the CRC Press Web site at www.crcpress.com

Library of Congress Card Number 00-031433
Visit the Taylor & Francis Web site at
http://www.taylorandfrancis.com

and the CRC Press Web site at
http://www.crcpress.com

Preface

The title of this book, *Drug Synergism and Dose-Effect Data Analysis*, could just as well be reversed to, *Dose-Effect Data Analysis and Drug Synergism*. The two topics are inextricably woven and both are covered in this book. I decided on the first title because synergism, as a quantitative topic, has been neglected in mainstream textbooks of pharmacology, though the term and its synonyms, *potentiation* and *superadditivity*, are mentioned frequently. As used here, these terms refer to a phenomenon characterized by drug combinations that produce exaggerated effects. These effects can be the intended effects or the adverse effects of a combination of drugs or other chemicals. In some sense, all pharmacologists, physicians, and most other scientists know what synergism is, yet, it seems, few are familiar with the quantitative methodology that is needed to differentiate synergistic responses from the simply additive responses that are the "expected" effects of drug combinations. The distinction is a quantitative one, and this book deals with the quantitative methodology that is needed to make this distinction. Even when a single drug is administered it enters a system containing myriads of other chemicals and, therefore, interaction with one or more of these compounds is possible. Thus, in a very real sense, this topic has broad applications.

The mathematical foundation for studying the effects of chemical combinations was laid in the first half of the twentieth century, mainly through the works of Fisher, Gaddum, Bliss, and Finney. Much of that early work was directed toward the joint action of various toxins, insecticides, and fungicides. Probit analysis, a powerful method for analyzing quantal dose-effect data, grew out of that early work which almost always used models that constrained the (log) dose-effect data of the individual drugs to yield parallel regression lines. That constraint, the intrinsic complexity of the probit method, and the absence of computers in that era probably contributed to the present-day neglect of this old literature and, thus, its exclusion in the curricula of today's students of pharmacology and toxicology. The current wide-spread availability of computers, a broadening of the theory, and a general recognition of the importance of combinations in modern pharmacology have restored interest in this subject. This expanded theory and the many old and new calculation algorithms it uses constitute the main subject of this book, and numerous examples illustrate these calculations.

When experiments are planned, the investigator must have some expectation of the kind of data that may result and, hence, a familiarity with the methodology needed to analyze the data. This is an important part of experimental design. In drug experiments these methods must take into account the variability that is expressed in the data collected. Indeed, the abundance of experimental designs, the many ways of measuring effects, and the never-ending appearance of new drugs and chemicals underscore the need to deal with this variability. Hence, much of the material of this book draws on statistics. Statistical methods, and the theory that underlies these statistics, come from observations of dose-response data and the model curves and equations that describe these data. Therefore, many topics in this book deal with dose-effect data, starting with observations from a single drug and expanding the concepts to more than one drug and the effects that result from such combinations.

Our emphasis is always quantitative since the problem of distinguishing a super-additive response from an additive (expected) response is intrinsically quantitative. When synergism is observed, is it dependent on the *doses* of the respective drugs, or on the *ratio of doses* in the combination, or on the *measurement system* that describes the effect? All of these questions must be ultimately answered, even though in most cases the mechanism responsible for the synergism may still remain unknown. But identifying synergism is, in itself, a valuable first step in illuminating the mechanism.

This book's first three chapters deal mainly with dose-response relations, the statistical analysis of the data that come from these relations, and the models that describe them. Linear regression theory is an important part of this analysis. That topic, though well represented in many textbooks, is treated here with the special needs of the pharmacologist in mind. These include calculations of D_{50} (and *ED50*) values and their standard errors, relative potency determinations, and the common transformations of drug data that allow these estimates. In Chapter 4 we put this all together in calculations of synergism for *graded* data. Those calculations allow a distinction between synergism and additivity at one particular effect level. This idea is broadened in Chapter 5 where we discuss a newer concept, the *composite additive line*, that extends the analysis to other effect levels. Of special importance in pharmacology is the use of probit analysis, a subject that is absent in most statistics books. Probit analysis is a useful and powerful weighted regression technique that is ideally suited to drug experiments that produce binary outcomes (quantal effects) as opposed to effects on a continuous scale. Logit analysis, also applicable to quantal data, is also presented, and the pros and cons of both methods are discussed. Synergism, and the methodology that distinguishes it from simple additivity, has been traditionally tied to the *isobologram*. This historical plot, while useful for graphical display, does not lead to precise statistical conclusions. In that regard we have introduced an alternate graphical method (Chapter 7) that is more useful.

Much of the content of Chapters 7–11 is new. Especially noteworthy is the use of a single compound administered at two different anatomical sites. Site-site synergism represents a novel way of studying drug mechanisms and some of its benefits are discussed in Chapter 9. Also noteworthy is the *response surface* approach. In contrast to the isobolar approach that is tied to one effect level, this method examines interactions over a range of effects and doses.

As previously mentioned computer technology has had an important impact on the analysis of drug data. Some topics, such as probit analysis and nonlinear regression, admittedly require tedious calculations; prior to the widespread availability of computers these calculations taxed the ability and time of most scientists. Today, these calculations are readily performed with the aid of computers. However, the concepts behind these calculations still remain hidden. For that reason we have included material on nonlinear regression that is applicable to dose-response curves (in Chapter 11) and the details of probit analysis (in Chapter 6). With the exception of these two topics, virtually all the other calculations described in this book can be readily performed with the aid of a calculator and the Appendix tables, though many will still want the convenience of the computer. For that reason, a companion software package that performs the calculations is currently in preparation (see page 204). *Illustrations of calculations in the text use fewer figures than those retained by the computer. Accordingly, some intermediate results in the text may differ slightly from computer values due to rounding.*

While our focus is on drug data, the methods presented are equally applicable to a wider class of chemicals, as is evident in the historical development of this subject. The works of many scientists inspired me to write this book. Most notable are those "giants" of pharmacology and statistics, previously mentioned, who paved the way over 50 years ago. But a special thanks is also due to all those scientists whose works are cited throughout this book, especially Martin Adler, Alan Cowan, Donna Hammond, Frank Porreca, Robert Raffa, Sandra Roerig, and George Wilcox. I am also much indebted to Jeffrey McCary who wrote the companion computer programs and my editor, Bob Stern, who encouraged me to undertake this work and Helena Redshaw who kept things running smoothly. Steve Menke deserves special thanks for his excellent work in production. Finally, I would like to thank my family for excusing me from many family functions, basketball games, and track meets while I worked on this book.

R.J. Tallarida
Philadelphia
2000

The Author

Ronald J. Tallarida earned the B.S. and M.S. degrees in physics/mathematics and a Ph.D. in pharmacology. His primary appointment is as Professor of Pharmacology at Temple University School of Medicine, Philadelphia; he also serves as Adjunct Professor of Biomedical Engineering (mathematics) at Drexel University in Philadelphia where he started his professional career. Dr. Tallarida received the Lindback Award for Distinguished Teaching while in the Drexel mathematics department. He is the author of the popular *Pocket Book of Integrals and Mathematics Formulas,* currently in its third edition, also published by CRC/Chapman & Hall.

As an author and researcher, Dr. Tallarida has published over 200 works, including eight books, and is a frequent consultant to both industry and government agencies for his quantitative work in theoretical pharmacology, data analysis, and combination drug studies. His research on drug synergism has been sponsored by the National Institute on Drug Abuse and by several pharmaceutical firms.

Contents

To

Christopher
R.J.
and
Theresa

CHAPTER 1

Combinations of Chemicals

I often say that when you can measure what you are speaking about, and express it in numbers, you know something about it; but when you cannot express it in numbers, your knowledge is of a meagre and unsatisfactory kind; it may be the beginning of knowledge, but you have scarcely, in your thoughts, advanced to that stage of Science, whatever the matter my be.

Lord Kelvin (1824–1907)

1.1   Introduction

A drug or other chemical may produce multiple effects in the system with which it interacts. A system is a set of interconnected components that has some purpose. In biology the system is often an entire organism. But other systems may be considered, such as an organ, a part of an organ, a cell, or a cellular component. An effect is a change in some attribute of the system. If the chemical is a fertilizer an obvious effect is the change in crop yield. If the chemical is a pesticide the effect might be the destruction or inhibition of the invading pest. In a biomedical context the chemicals of most interest in this book are drugs and endogenous compounds, and the effects are changes in the organism or part thereof. Familiar effects of drugs include changes in blood pressure, body temperature, heart rate, pain perception, etc. These are overt effects; other drug effects are intimate and not easily observed, such as the opening or closing of an ion channel in the cell membrane or the release of some other chemical substance from the cell. Drug effects can be desirable or undesirable (adverse effects). The main concern of this book is the study of two or more chemicals present together. Specifically, the interest is in drugs or other chemicals that act together to produce overtly similar effects, e.g., two analgesics or two antihypertensives.

When compounds with similar overt actions are present together, the combined effect may be predictable from knowledge of the individual drug potencies, i.e., there is simple additivity. In contrast, the effect of the combination may be either exaggerated or even attenuated. The exaggerated effect is termed *super-additive* or *synergistic* whereas the blunted effect is termed *sub-additive*. In each of these cases the individual compounds are contributing to the effect, but something occurs with their joint presence that either enhances or diminishes the effect expected from the pair.

Whether the pair of compounds consists of drugs, fertilizers, pesticides, or any other chemical types that act similarly, the methods of analysis presented here will apply. Our focus is on the relation between concentrations and effects and the methodology that distinguishes between additive and non-additive interactions, but, in some cases, this distinction may also help us better understand the intimate actions of the compounds. Several methods of analysis for distinguishing between simple additivity and the other non-additive outcomes will be discussed. These involve the use of quantitative information regarding the dose (or concentration) and the magnitude of the effect. The data contributing to this information are analyzed in a variety of different ways, very often from graphs of the relation between concentration and effect or from suitable mathematical transformations of these quantities. Accordingly, the dose-response relation is a key topic that is applied throughout this book.

Drug effects are often highly variable and the variability exhibited in this kind of data necessitates the use of statistical methodology. Thus, much of the material we discuss will consist of dose-effect curves and the statistical analysis of these curves, often with the aim of distinguishing simple additivity from sub-additivity and synergism for compounds acting together. Synergism is especially important in clinical situations with drugs, for it allows the use of smaller amounts of the constituent drugs. An adverse effect may also synergize, a phenomenon of special importance in clinical situations. The detection of synergism may also be useful in illuminating mechanisms of drug action and in the development of new theories. The same applies to synergistic combinations of other classes of chemicals. Although observational results are the primary material of pharmacology, the use of theory allows a correlation of these results, places them into the regularities of experience that we call principles, and uses these principles to predict the results of new experiments.

1.2   Independent joint action of drugs

If the dose-response relation is known for each of two chemicals used individually, how can the expected response for some combination of the two be calculated? This is a key question that was first systematically addressed by Bliss (1939) and subsequently expanded by Finney (1942) in connection with insecticides. An important consideration is whether the two chemicals act independently. Bliss referred to three types of joint action that he termed *independent joint action, similar joint action* and *synergistic action*. An important concept contained in the first two of these is the idea of independent action. Similar and independent action are useful for our future discussion of drug combinations. By this we mean that each drug produces overtly similar effects (for example, each lowers blood pressure) such that all or part of one component may be substituted for the other in some proportion that is based on the dose-response relations of the two.

For example, an antihypertensive drug that lowers blood pressure by blocking angiotensin II receptors and one that exerts its antihypertensive effect through diuresis would fit this definition of similar independent joint action. Their individual potencies allow a calculation of how much of one is equivalent to the other in the production of this effect, a calculation that is discussed in the next section. In contrast, two antihypertensive drugs that have general *beta* adrenoceptor block as components of their action would not fit this definition because of competition of the two for the common *beta* receptor.

In general, if two overtly similar drugs (either two antagonists or two agonists) act on the same cellular receptor, their actions are not independent because the effect of their combination depends on the bound concentrations of the two (and their intrinsic activities if they are agonists). One could not substitute an amount of one for the other in a combination based solely on their individual dose-response relations because a change in the concentration of one affects the bound concentrations of both. (Competition is discussed in Chapter 9.) The importance of independent action is further illustrated in our discussion of additivity as it is commonly defined in pharmacology.

1.3   Additivity

Drugs or other chemicals that produce overtly similar effects will generally do so with different doses. The dose-response relation of each agent provides this information and allows one to focus on a specific magnitude of the effect. For example, two drugs that are each capable of increasing the heart rate may differ in the respective doses needed to increase the rate. To distinguish these quantitatively one can choose an effect level, for example a rate increase of 10 beats per minute. The first drug might achieve this with a dose of 100 mg whereas the second requires only 25 mg. These are indicators of drug *potency*. The drug that requires the lower dose is said to have a greater potency than the other. The dose ratio, in this case 100/25 = 4, called the *relative potency*, is a convenient indicator of this quantitative attribute of the drug pair. This same relative potency may or may not apply to all levels of effect for these two drugs, a concept that is discussed in some detail in Chapter 2. For now we will assume a constant relative potency, i.e., one drug is four times more potent than the other at *all levels of effect* achieved by each drug. Further, we now introduce notations that will be convenient in this and in subsequent discussions.

For drug A, the lower potency drug, its dose when it acts alone is denoted by the italicized symbol, A; for drug B, the corresponding quantity is denoted B. The relative potency R is then A/B, a value greater than one. We now consider the situation in which both drugs are present together. In this situation lower case symbols are used, i.e., we denote by a and b the doses of the respective constituents when given as a combination. Because these drugs are assumed to have a constant relative potency (R) the combination (a, b) can be expressed as an equivalent quantity of either drug. If drug A is the reference drug then the combination dose satisfies the relation

$$a + Rb = A. \qquad (1.1)$$

In words, Equation 1.1 means that one can use respective amounts a and b calculated from the above in order to achieve the effect of dose A of drug A acting alone. Implicit in Equation 1.1 is the concept of independent joint action, i.e., the presence of B is like the addition of a more concentrated form of A. The same combination (a, b) can also be expressed in terms of an equivalent of drug B and is given by the equation

$$a/R + b = B. \qquad (1.2)$$

Here the less potent drug (A) acts like a dilute version of the other and adds to B. The relations expressed by Equations 1.1 and 1.2 mean that the doses in the combination contribute to the effect in accord with the individual drug potencies, a situation that is termed *additive*. Rearrangement of these gives a more familiar form:

$$a/A + b/B = 1. \qquad (1.3)$$

In each of the above equations, the doses A and B are equieffective doses of the individual agents when each is present alone, R is the ratio A/B, and the quantities a and b are the respective doses in the combination that give the effect level achieved by dose A alone or dose B alone. When the relative potency R is the same at all effect levels the first two forms are convenient; however, when R varies with the effect level, the more explicit relation of Equation 1.3 is convenient because it uses the values of A and B that apply to that effect. Equieffective dose pairs are termed *isoboles*; thus, $(A, 0)$, $(0, B)$ and the pair (a, b) given by the above relations are isoboles. Additivity as defined here is a most important concept. Departure from additivity means that some kind of interaction occurs when both substances are present together. Hence, calculating quantities that are additive is the basis for determining these departures when actual pairs are studied. Nonadditive pairs may be a useful first step in illuminating mechanisms.

1.4   Isobologram

Equation 1.3 provides a simple graph of equieffective dose pairs (a, b). If A and B are known to be the respective doses that give a specified effect, e.g., 50% of the maximum effect, when each agent acts alone then these are constants that are used to identify the doses a and b in a combination that produces this same effect. These combination doses must satisfy Equation 1.3. For example, if $A = 500$ mg and $B = 100$ mg, then the equation, $a/500 + b/100 = 1$, gives additive dose combinations such as $(100, 80)$, $(250, 50)$, etc. The totality of pairs (a, b) graph as the straight line shown in Figure 1.1. This *line of additivity* has Cartesian coordinates that represent all possible combinations that are equivalent in producing the effect of either 500 mg of drug A or 100 mg of drug B. A graph of this kind is useful for displaying the results of actual tests with combinations. Such testing may reveal departures from additivity. Suppose, for example, that the combination $a = 100$ mg, $b = 50$ mg produced the specified effect level. This point $(100, 50)$ lies below the line of additivity as shown in Figure 1.2 as point P, meaning that lesser quantities of drugs A and B are needed in the combination. Some interaction has taken place,

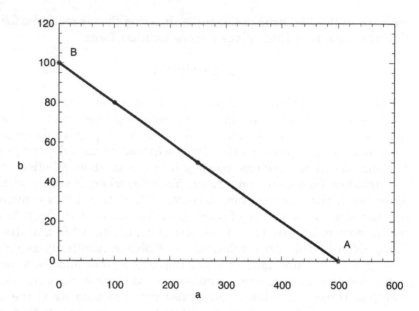

Figure 1.1. Line of additivity of the isobologram. Intercepts are doses of each when present alone.

either between the drugs or the systems on which they jointly act, and therefore quantities less than those predicted by additivity are needed. This is called a super-additive or *synergistic* combination. In contrast, some combinations may require doses that are greater than the additive amounts of Equation 1.3 in which case the point representing the combination will lie above the line of additivity as shown in Figure 1.2 as point **Q**. This phenomenon means sub-additivity, i.e., the constituents are somewhat antagonistic for some reason. This graph, consisting of the additive line and the actual dose pairs needed to attain the specific effect level is called an *isobologram*. It was introduced by Loewe who conducted a number of studies of combinations that used this kind of graph. (See Loewe, 1927, 1928, 1953, 1957.) These non-additive cases are expressed as inequality relations that contrast with Equation 1.3 as follows:

$$a/A + b/B < 1. \tag{1.4}$$

$$a/A + b/B > 1. \tag{1.5}$$

Relation 1.4 indicates synergism or super-additivity whereas Relation 1.5 means sub-additivity.

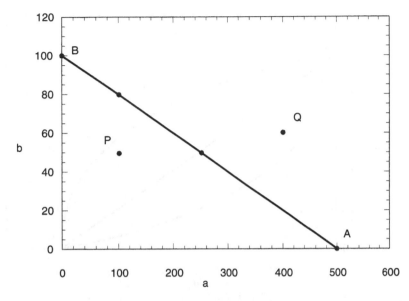

Figure 1.2. Isobologram showing line of additivity and dose combination P that is synergistic and dose combination Q that is sub-additive.

Testing two drugs together may reveal many synergistic combinations, and, thus, their graphical representation suggests a smooth curve that is concave upward as shown in Figure 1.3 (curve I) or a curve that is concave downward, indicative of sub-additive combinations, shown as curve II in the figure. Curves, or sets of discrete points (doses) that give the same effect, are termed *isoboles*; these are curves of constant effect and have termini (axial points) that indicate the individual doses, *A* of drug A and *B* of drug B when each is present alone. Although smooth curves such as these indicate either synergism or sub-additivity over all dose combinations, there is no reason why such patterns must occur when actual combinations of chemicals are tested. In other words, some dose pairs may be synergistic while others are additive, or even sub-additive. Accordingly, the isoboles of Figure 1.3 should be regarded only as models that could describe the combined action of two active drugs.

An interesting case is that in which one of the drugs (drug A) is inactive when given alone. Here the isobole of additivity is a horizontal line (Figure 1.4) so that synergism and sub-additivity are indicated by dose pairs giving points P and Q below and above this line, respectively.

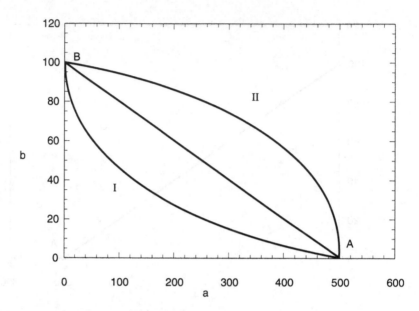

Figure 1.3. Isobologram showing line of additivity and curves for combinations that are synergistic (curve I) and sub-additive (curve II).

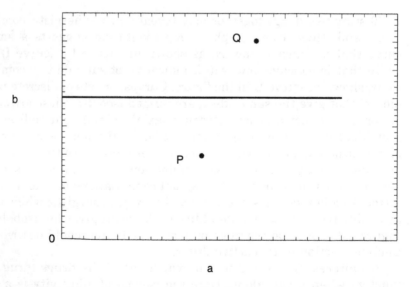

Figure 1.4. Isobologram when one drug (A) is inactive. The active drug (B) produces the desired effect with dose b and this effect is independent of the dose of A in a theoretically additive combination. If actual dose combinations, indicated by points P and Q, produce the specified effect, these are synergistic and sub-additive, respectively.

1.5   Chloral hydrate and ethyl alcohol

The isobologram seems to have attracted little attention until it was used in a well-publicized study of the combined action of chloral hydrate and alcohol by Gessner and Cabana (1970). Both agents are hypnotics; that is, they are capable of inducing sleep, and this study was aimed at answering the question of whether the combination of the two was synergistic. The experiment was carried out in mice that received intraperitoneal doses of the individual drugs and combinations. An indicator of hypnosis was the loss of the righting reflex and that could be quantitated for each dose or dose combination as the proportion of animals that displayed this endpoint. The effect level used was hypnosis in 50% of the mice tested ($p = 0.5$). The dose of either drug (acting alone) that gives this level is the *ED50*. For ethanol (horizontal axis) the *ED50* was found to be 2666 mg/kg, and for chloral hydrate the value was 244 mg/kg (vertical axis). These are the respective mean values obtained from analysis of the individual dose-effect curves of the agents. For our current purpose, we will postpone discussions of dose-effect data analysis and the methods that gave these estimates of the means and thus concentrate only on the display of data points shown on the isobologram of Figure 1.5.

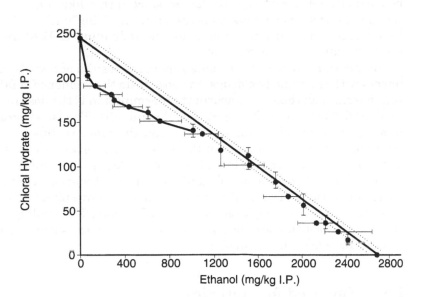

Figure 1.5. Isobologram for the hypnotic effect of a combination of ethyl alcohol and chloral hydrate. (From Gessner and Cabana, A study of the hypnotic and of the toxic effects of chloral hydrate and ethanol, *J. Pharmacol. Exp. Ther.*, 1970, with permission.)

This figure shows a solid line having vertical intercept 244 and horizontal intercept 2666, these being the individual drug *ED50* values. This is the line of *additivity*. Individual dose pairs that gave 50% effects are also plotted, and these points show either horizontal or vertical error bars whose meaning is related to the way these were obtained. In some cases the chloral hydrate dose was fixed, and the amount of ethanol used concurrently to produce the 50%·response was estimated (from regression analysis). Accordingly, this estimate of the ethanol mean dose has statistical confidence limits that are displayed as horizontal bars through the points. In cases in which ethanol was fixed and chloral hydrate varied until the 50% response was attained, we get estimates of the latter's dose and the confidence limits of this mean are indicated by vertical bars.

The main idea here is that some of the data points appear to be well off the line of additivity, while others are close to the line and have error bars that intersect it. As a purely visual conclusion this means that some combinations are synergistic whereas others are simply additive. In other words, synergism is not only a property of the drug pair but also depends on the relative amounts in the combination tested. Another observation is that a plot of this kind may not be adequate for a rigorous conclusion since terms like "on" and "off" the line are loose constructs, as is the location of the "line" itself, since its vertical and horizontal intercepts (the individual *ED50s*) are also estimates and, thus, have error.

In this same article the authors report the results of toxicity experiments with the same two drugs. In those tests the incidence of fatality was determined; thus, the important determination is the dose (or dose combination) that is lethal in 50% of the animals. The isobologram in this case was based on *LD50* values and therefore is different from the isobologram for hypnosis. In the lethality isobologram (not shown here), there was synergism for only one of the dose pairs tested (highest ratio of chloral hydrate), simple additivity in combinations containing lower proportions of chloral hydrate, and apparent sub-additivity in combinations containing larger amounts of alcohol. This finding points out that the isobologram for one endpoint is not necessarily the same as that for some other endpoint.

1.6   The need for statistics

The distinction between additive and nonadditive actions uses dose values that produce a specified level of effect. Up to now our discussion has treated these doses as exact quantities. These are displayed as points on the isobologram, and the basis of this plot is the additivity equation given by Equation 1.3 and the inequalities given in expressions 1.4 and 1.5. But in each of these expressions the quantities, a, b, A, and B that denote doses, represent values that are known only in a probabilistic sense. In other words the values for these quantities are only estimates made from dose-effect data. This is so because of the inherent variability of the dose-effect data so that the quantities are dose (or concentration) values that are derived from modeling these data.

In practice, dose-effect data are displayed as points on a graph. For any given drug or chemical, the administration of even a precise dose leads to different measures of the effect, whether in the same animal (or system) or in different animals treated identically. These different outcomes may be due in part to problems in the metric used to define the effect, but, even in the absence of metric problems, there is inherent biological variability. How, then, are the doses a, b, etc., obtained? Most often these come from the mathematical models that are used to describe the underlying relation between dose and effect. Thus, a precisely controlled dose leads to a variable response and some method (such as "least squares") is used to obtain the mean effect. Commonly, regression methods are used to estimate the mean effect. The techniques of regression analysis (linear and nonlinear) require that the dose (independent variable) be error free and that the effect values obey some statistical distribution. In practical terms there is error in the dependent variable (the effect); it follows, therefore, that the use of models carries with it some uncertainty.

Since the true effect of a dose is unknown and merely estimated from the dose-response curve, the assignment of a value to it, e.g., 50% of the animals tested, means that the dose is also an estimate from the model equation. A theoretical effect level is used in the derived model equation, and the dose is calculated from this equation. In short, these calculated doses also have errors, even though the actual doses used as data in the model are presumed to be error free. Thus, every $ED50$ or $LD50$ is an estimate, a number with confidence limits. When these values are used for the individual drugs as intercept numbers defining the line of additivity in an isobologram, it becomes clear that the precise location of this line is unknown, i.e., the values of A and B used to anchor the line are random variables that often have wide confidence limits. This is also true for the combination doses (a, b) so that all constituents of the isobologram have errors.

If modeling is done on the isobolar points (a, b), there is the additional theoretical problem of dealing with uncertainty in both variables. For example, the common linear regression procedure (discussed in Chapters 2 and 3) would not apply to this situation of dual uncertainty. The isobologram is thus a visual display that has some utility in approximate analysis but is not very useful as a sole device for making precise conclusions about the nature of the interaction, i.e., distinguishing between additive and nonadditive joint action.

Special caution is needed in situations in which the points appear somewhat close to the "line" of additivity. Much of the material of this book deals with methods of analysis that allow statistical tests to distinguish departures from simple additivity, and, because the underlying theory incorporates doses such as $a, b, A,$ and B, we shall devote the next two chapters to discussions of how these estimates are made from dose-effect data analysis. The reader who is sufficiently well versed in this topic can skip these chapters and go on to Chapter 4, which deals with methods that distinguish synergism (and sub-additivity) from additivity in common experimental designs.

1.7   The emergence of quantitative methods for studying drug combinations

Quantitative methodology for studying biologically active chemical combinations began with applications to poisons. The method of isoboles had its earliest application in studies of data from toxicity tests for the assay of insecticides and fungicides, and that application, in turn, led to broader pharmacological uses and new statistical developments. Yet, quantitative methods for studying agonist combinations have not been prominently featured in mainstream textbooks of pharmacology. Nevertheless, in recent years the importance of this subject has been appreciated by more and more pharmacologists, especially those who study drugs that affect the nervous system to alter pain perception, behavior, locomotion, and mood. Indeed, these are also the classes of drugs that tend to be abused, and this recognition probably accounts for the growing use of isobolographic and related quantitative methods by investigators in the drug abuse field. It is well known that drug abusers rarely abuse one drug; most often poly-drug usage is the norm.

Properly used drugs also interact, thereby enhancing both the desirable and the undesirable effects. Aside from the obvious clinical importance there is a growing recognition that the quantitative study of drug combinations, especially the detection of true drug synergism, can be a useful first step in illuminating the mechanism. Many recent drug combination studies, especially those dealing with opioids and other analgesics, have this as their major goal. This broadened application has, in turn, spawned new statistical developments to aid in this effort.

The reference list at the end of this chapter includes a number of studies that employed these methods and thus illustrate the use of theory and statistics. The list also includes works that are primarily concerned with theory and statistics. These are useful for improving experimental design and data analysis. While this reference list is not exhaustive it does provide a guide for investigators who wish to undertake quantitative studies of drug combinations. Many of these references are cited specifically in the detailed subjects contained in subsequent chapters of this book.

CHAPTER 1

References and Suggested Reading

S denotes works that are primarily statistical and/or theoretical.

Adams, J.U., Tallarida, R.J., Geller, E.B., and Adler, M.W. Combinations of PL017 and DPDPE produce simple additivity in an analgesic test in rats: An isobolographic analysis. In *Problems of Drug Dependence*, L.S. Harris, Ed. NIDA Research Monograph 119:301, 1992.

Adams, J.U., Tallarida, R.J., Geller, E.B., and Adler, M.W. Isobolographic super-additivity between delta and *mu* opioid agonists in the rat depends on the ratio of compounds, the *mu* agonist and the analgesic assay used. *J. Pharmacol. Exp. Ther.* 266:1261–1267, 1993.

Aran, S. and Hammond, D.L. Antagonism of baclofen-induced antinociception by intrathecal administration of phaclofen or 2–hydroxy-saclofen, but not delta-aminovaleric acid in the rat. *J. Pharmacol. Exp. Ther.* 257:360–368, 1991.

Berenbaum, M.C. What is Synergy? *Pharmacol. Rev.* 41:93–144, 1989. **(S)**

Bian, D., Ossipov, M.H., Ibrahim, M., Raffa, R.B., Tallarida, R.J., Malan, T.P., Lai, J., and Porreca, F. Loss of antiallodynic and antinociceptive spinal-supraspinal morphine synergy in nerve-injured rats: Restoration by MK-801 or dynorphin antiserum. *Brain Res.* 831:55–63, 1999.

Bliss, C.I. The method of probits. *Science*, 79: 38–39, 1934. **(S)**

Bliss, C.I. The method of probits — a correction. *Science*, 79: 409–410, 1934. **(S)**

Bliss, C.I. The determination of dosage-mortality curves for small numbers. *Quart. J. Pharmacol.* 11:192–216, 1938. **(S)**

Bliss, C.I. The toxicity of poisons applied jointly. *Ann. Appl. Biol.* 26:585–615, 1939.**(S)**

Busby, R.C and Tallarida, R.J. On the analysis of straight line data in pharmacology and biochemistry. *J. Theor. Biol.* 93:867–879, 1981. **(S)**

Carter, W.H., Gennings, C., Staniswalis, J.C., Campbell, E.D., and White, K.L., Jr. A statistical approach to the construction and analysis of isobolograms. *J. Am. Coll. Toxicol.* 7:963–973, 1988. **(S)**

Draper, N. and Smith, H. *Applied Regression Analysis,* 2nd ed. Wiley, New York, 1981. **(S)**

Eisenstein, T.K., Meissler, J.J., Tallarida, R.J., Rogers, T.J., Geller, E., and Adler M.W. Combination of opioids with selectivity for mu or delta receptors exhibit dose-dependent super- and sub-additive effects on splenic plaque-forming cell responses. (Abstract) *Soc. Leukocyte Biol.*, Baltimore, Dec., 1997.

Fairbanks, C.A. and Wilcox, G.L. Spinal antinociceptive synergism between morphine and clonidine persists in mice made acutely or chronically tolerant to morphine. *J. Pharmacol. Exp. Ther.* 288:1107–1116, 1999.

Fieller, E.C. A fundamental formula in the statistics of biological assay and some applications. *Quart. J. Pharmacy and Pharmacol.* 17:117–123, 1944. **(S)**

Finney, D.J. The analysis of toxicity tests on mixtures of poisons. *Ann. Appl. Biol.* 29:82–94, 1942. **(S)**

Finney, D.J. *Probit Analysis*, 3rd ed. Cambridge, 1971. **(S)**

Fisher, R.A. Appendix to Bliss, C.I. The case of zero survivors. *Ann. Appl. Biol.* 22: 164–165, 1935. **(S)**

Freeman, K.A., Bove, A.A., and Tallarida, R.J. Additive and super-additive combinations of diltiazem and glyceryl trinitrate in isolated rabbit aorta. *Drug Dev. Res.* 25: 171–179, 1992.

Gaddum, J. H. Reports on biological standards, III. Methods of biological assay depending on a quantal response. *Spec. Rep. Ser. Med. Res. Council*, London, no. 183, 1933. **(S)**

Gennings, C, Carter, W.H., Jr., Campbell, E.D., Staniswalis, J.G., Martin, T.J., Martin, B.R., and White, K.L., Jr., Isobolographic characterization of drug interactions incorporating biological variability. *J. Pharmacol. Exp. Ther.* 252:208–217, 1990. **(S)**

Gentili, M., Houssel, P., Osman, M., Henel, D., Juhel, A., and Bonnet, F. Intraarticular morphine and clonidine produce comparable analgesia but the combination is not more effective. *Br. J. Anaesth.* 79:660–661, 1997.

Gessner, P.K. The isobolographic method applied to drug interactions. In *Drug Interactions*, Morselli, P.L., Garattini, S., and Cohen, S.N., Eds. Raven Press, New York, 1974.

Gessner, P.K. and Cabana, B.E. A study of the hypnotic and of the toxic effects of chloral hydrate and ethanol. *J. Pharmacol. Exp. Ther.* 174: 247–259, 1970.

Hammond, D.L., Donahue, B.B., and Stewart, P.E. Role of spinal delta-1 and delta-2 opioid receptors in the antinociception produced by microinjection of L-glutamate in the ventromedial medulla of the rat. *Brain Res.* 765:177–181, 1997.

Hammond, D.L., Hurley, R.W., Glabow, T.S., and Tallarida, R.J. Characterization of the interaction between supraspinal and spinal delta-1 and delta-2 opioid receptors in the production of antinociception in the rat. (Abstract) *Soc. Neurosci.* 1998.

Hewlett, P.S. and Plackett, R.L. *The Interpretation of Quantal Responses in Biology.* University Park Press, Baltimore, 1979. **(S)**

Horan, P., Tallarida, R.J., Haaseth, R.C., Matsunaga, T.O., Hruby, V.J., and Porreca, F. Antinociceptive interactions of opioid delta receptor agonists with morphine in mice: Supra- and sub-additivity. *Life Sci.* 50: 1535–1541, 1992.

Hurley, R.W., Grabow, T.S. Tallarida, R.J., and Hammond, D.L. Interaction between medullary and spinal delta-1 and delta-2 opioid receptors in the production of antinociception in the rat. *J. Pharmacol. Exp. Ther.* 289:993–999, 1999.

Kimmel, H.L., Tallarida, R.J., and Holtzman, S.G. Synergism between buprenorphine and cocaine on the rotational behavior of the nigrally-lesioned rat. *Psychopharmacology.* 133:372–377, 1997.

Lashbrook, J., Ossipov, M.H., Hunter, J.C., Raffa, R.B., Tallarida, R.J., and Porreca, F. Synergistic antiallodynic effects of spinal morphine with ketorollac and selective COX-1 and COX-2 inhibitors in nerve-injured rats. *Pain* 82:65–72, 1999.

Lee, N.M., Leybin, L., Chang, J.K., and Loh, H.H. Opiate and peptide interaction: Effect of enkephalins on morphine analgesia. *Eur. J. Pharmacol.* 68: 181, 1980.

Loewe, S. Die Mischiarnei. *Klin. Wochenschr.* 6:1077–1085, 1927. **(S)**

Loewe, S. Die quantitativen Probleme der Pharmakologie. *Ergebn. Physiol.* 27:47–187, 1928. **(S)**

Loewe, S. The problem of synergism and antagonism of combined drugs. *Arzneimittelforschung* 3:285–290, 1953. **(S)**

Loewe, S. Antagonism and antagonists. *Pharmacol. Rev.* 9:237–242, 1957. **(S)**

Mattia, A., Vanderah, T., Raffa, R.B., Vaught, J.L., Tallarida, R.J., and Porreca, F. Characterization of the unusual antinociceptive profile of tramadol in mice. *Drug Dev. Res.* 28:176–182, 1992.

McCary, J.D. and Tallarida, R.J. A program for analyzing synergistic interactions from dose-effect data. *Analgesia* 3:297–305, 1998. **(S)**

McGowan, M.K. and Hammond, D.L. Intrathecal GABA-B antagonists attenuate the antinociception produced by microinjection of L-glutamate into the ventromedial medulla of the rat. *Brain Res.* 607:39–46, 1993.

Ossipov, M.H., Harris, S., Lloyd, P., and Messineo, E. An isobolographic analysis of the antinociceptive effect of systemically and intrathecally administered combinations of clonidine and opiates. *J. Pharmacol. Exp. Ther.* 255:1107–1116, 1990.

Ossipov, M.H., Lozito, R., Messineo, E., Green, J., Harris, S., and Lloyd, P. Spinal antinociceptive synergy between clonidine and morphine, U69593, and DPDPE: Isobolographic analysis. *Life Sci.* 46:PL71–76, 1990

Pircio, A.W., Buyniski, J.P., and Roebel, L.E. Pharmacological effects of a combination of butorphanol and acetaminophen. *Arch. Int. Pharmacodyn.* 235:116–123, 1978.

Plummer, J.L. and Short, T.G. Statistical modeling of the effects of drug combinations. *J. Pharmacol. Methods.* 23:297–309, 1990. **(S)**

Porreca, F., Jiang, Qi, and Tallarida, R.J. Modulation of morphine antinoci-
ception by peripheral [Leu5]-enkephalin: A synergistic interaction. *Eur. J. Pharmacol.* 179: 463–468, 1990.

Porreca, F., Mosberg, H.I., Hurst, R., Hruby, V.J., and Burks, T.J. Roles of mu, delta and kappa opioid receptors in spinal and supraspinal mediation of gastrointestinal transit effects and hot plate analgesia in the mouse. *J. Pharmacol. Exp. Ther.* 230: 341–348, 1984.

Price, D.D., Mao, J., Juan, L., Caruso, F.S., Frenk, H., and Mayer, D.J. Effects of the combined oral administration of NSAIDS and dextromethorphan on behavioral symptoms indicative of arthritic pain in rats. *Pain* 68:119–127, 1996.

Raffa, R.B., Friderichs, E., Reimann, W., Shank, R.P., Codd, E.E., Vaught, J.L., Jacoby, H.I., and Selve, N. Complementary and synergistic antinoci-ceptive interaction between the enantiomers of tramadol. *J. Pharmacol. Exp. Ther.* 267:331–340, 1993.

Raffa, R.B., Stone, D.J., and Tallarida, R.J. Antinociceptive self synergy between spinal and supraspinal acetaminophen (Paracetamol). International Pain Conference Austria, 1999.

Roerig, S.C., Hoffman, R.G., Takemori, A.E., Wilcox, G.L., and Fujimoto, J.M. Isobolographic analysis of analgesic interactions between intrathecally and intracerebroventricularly administered fentanyl, morphine and D-Ala^2-D-Leu-Enkephalin in morphine-tolerant and nontolerant mice. *J. Pharmacol. Exp. Ther.* 257:1091–1099, 1991.

Sofuoglo, M., Portoghese, P.S., and Takemori, A.E. Differential antagonism of delta opioid agonists by naltrindole and its benzofuran analog (NTB) in mice: Evidence for delta receptor subtypes. *J. Pharmacol. Exp. Ther.* 257:676–680, 1991.

Tallarida, R.J. Statistical analysis of drug combinations for synergism. *Pain* 49:93–97, 1992. **(S)**

Tallarida, R.J. and Murray, R.B. *Manual of Pharmacologic Calculation with Computer Programs,* 2nd ed. Springer Verlag, New York, 1987. **(S)**

Tallarida, R.J. and Raffa, R.B. Testing for synergism over a range of fixed ratio drug combinations: Replacing the isobologram. *Life Sci.* 58:PL23–28, 1996. **(S)**

Tallarida, R.J., Kimmel, H.L and Holtzman, S.G. Theory and statistics of detecting synergism between two active drugs: Cocaine and buprenor-phine. *Psychopharmacology* 133:378–382, 1997. **(S)**

Tallarida, R.J., Porreca, F., and Cowan, A. Statistical analysis of drug-drug and site-site interactions with isobolograms. *Life Sci.* 45:947–961, 1989. **(S)**

Tallarida, R.J., Stone, D.J., and Raffa, R.B. Efficient designs for studying synergistic drug combinations. *Life Sci.* 61:PL417–425, 1997. **(S)**

Tallarida, R.J., Stone, D.J., McCary, J.D., and Raffa, R.B. A response surface analysis of synergism between morphine and clonidine. *J. Pharmacol. Exp. Ther.* 289:8–13, 1999. **(S)**

Wessinger, W.D. Approaches to the study of drug interactions in behavioral pharmacology. *Neurosci. Biobehav. Rev.* 10:103–113, 1986.

Wilcox, G.L., Carlsson, K.H., Jochim, A., and Jurna, I. Mutual potentiation of antinociceptive effects of morphine and clonidine on motor and sensory responses in rat spinal cord. *Brain Res.* 405:84–93, 1987.

Woolverton, W.L. Analysis of drug interactions in behavioral pharmacology. In *Neurobehavioral Pharmacology*, Thompson, T., Dews, P.B., and Barrett, J.E. Eds. Lawrence Erlbaum Assoc., Hillsdale, NJ 275–302, 1987.

Yeung, J.C. and Rudy, T.A. Multiplicative interactions between narcotic agonisms expressed at spinal and supraspinal sites of antinociceptive action as revealed by concurrent intrathecal and intracerebroventricular injections of morphine. *J. Pharmacol. Exp. Ther.* 215:633–642, 1980.

CHAPTER 2

Dose-Response Analysis

A drug-induced effect may be expressed on a continuous scale or on a binary scale. In many isolated tissue experiments, e.g., isolated muscle preparations, the effect is measured as the developed force, a continuous variable. In certain animal experiments the effect is the latency to display some endpoint and, thus, is measured as time. Both force and time are effects measured on a continuous scale. Examples of binary effects are hypnosis in an animal exhibited by the loss of the righting reflex, some well-defined motion, such as writhing, or death produced by some dose of the drug. In other words the event either occurs or does not occur. Both continuous and binary effects are used in the study of drug action and in describing the relation between the dose and the magnitude of the effect. Many theories have been proposed that attempt to explain how dose-effect data can be related to receptor events, and discussions of these theories may be found in several monographs (Ariens et al., 1964; Goldstein et al., 1974; Tallarida and Jacob, 1979; Tallarida et al., 1987; Kenakin, 1987; Lauffenburger and Linderman, 1993.) For our current purpose, the emphasis will be on the analysis of the data and not on the underlying receptor theory. In this regard, we shall begin with dose-effect data from effects measured on a continuous scale (such as time and force) as well as effects that can be reasonably approximated as continuous, such as the heart rate. When such effects are plotted against the dose or concentration of the drug (or chemical), a curve of some kind is used to model the data points, thereby producing a "graded" dose-effect curve. Chapter 6 is devoted to all-or-none (quantal) responses.

2.1   Efficacy and potency

Graded dose-effect data often exhibit certain features that allow statistical analysis and also provide concepts leading to definitions and notations that are useful in describing and analyzing data. In

Table 2.1. Dose-Response Data for Methoxamine HCl in Rabbit Aortic Strips

Conc. (M)	Force (mn)
1.40e-07	0.196
2.30e-07	0.588
4.10e-07	1.96
5.70e-07	3.33
8.00e-07	5.48
1.10e-06	7.84
1.50e-06	9.60
2.30e-06	12.5
3.90e-06	15.3
5.30e-06	16.8
8.00e-06	18.0
1.70e-05	19.2
4.20e-05	19.4

Strips of rabbit thoracic aorta, anchored to a force transducer, were placed in a Krebs bicarbonate muscle bath that was aerated with 95% O_2 + 5% CO_2. The drug was added with a pipette, allowed time to mix, and the equilibrium developed force (millinewtons) was recorded for each molar concentration. Data extracted from Raffa et al. (1979) and replotted in Figure 2.1.

Table 2.1, the drug is methoxamine HCl, and the effect is the change in isometric force that occurred in isolated aortic strips of the rabbit. The points are plotted in rectangular coordinates in Figure 2.1, and the graph shows several features that are common to many dose-effect curves. Effect increases as the dose is increased; hence, the effect is dose-related. Also, the effect is zero at the zero dose and rises to what appears to be a maximum; i.e., the effect is bounded from above by some value (in this case, 19.6 mn). This upper bound (or maximum) is a measure of the drug's *efficacy*. The efficacy of a particular drug or chemical, indicated by the maximum of its dose-effect curve, may be related to the maximum effect that can be attained by any known drug or other stimulus in this same preparation (the system maximum). The ratio of the drug maximum to the system maximum is thus a measure of the relative efficacy, a number that ranges from 0 to 1. *Agonists* are compounds with relative efficacy significantly greater than zero, and these are said to be *full* agonists or *strong* agonists if this measure is unity. Other chemicals that produce the same effect, but have lesser values of relative efficacy are termed *partial* agonists.

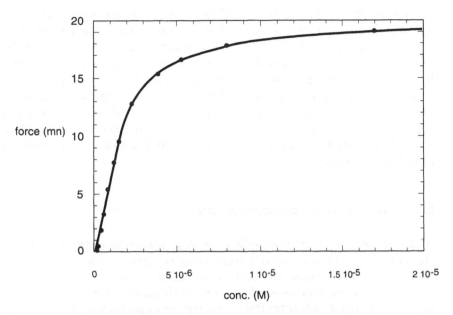

Figure 2.1. Methoxamine dose-response curve. (Redrawn from Raffa et al., 1979.)

While the measure of a drug's relative efficacy tells us something about its maximum effect, it gives no indication of how much of the drug is needed to attain this maximum or any other effect level. That kind of information is contained in the drug's dose-effect curve and is most conveniently summarized by a single number — a single dose that indicates the left-to-right position of the dose-effect curve. For this purpose, some effect level is needed as a reference. A common reference choice is an effect of magnitude equal to one half the system's maximum effect. With this choice of effect the dose is obtained from the smooth curve at the indicated half-maximal effect. This dose, taken from the curve, is a common measure of *potency*.

For two different drugs that attain the same maximum, such as two full agonists, these measures of potency provide a quantitative distinction. The drug that requires the lower dose to achieve the half-maximal effect is said to be more potent than the other. Equieffective doses (isoboles discussed in Chapter 1) are used in the analysis of drug combination data as previously described, and, very often, these are taken as the doses of the respective drugs that are required to attain the half maximal effect if both drugs attain the same maximum, such as two full agonists. When two drugs produce significantly different maximum effects, i.e., differ in efficacy, then equieffective doses can still be obtained from the dose-effect curve of each (as required in isobolar analysis), but clearly these will not be their respective half-maximal doses. Sometimes the effect of a drug or chemical is divided by its own maximum, thereby plotting a relative effect or percent of its own maximum. If this is done for each of two drugs with *different maxima,* one cannot easily obtain absolute equally effective doses from these curves alone since each would show a 100% response, but they are not indicative of the equal absolute effects that are needed in combination studies.

2.2   Doses and concentrations

Although we speak of dose-effect or dose-response data (and dose-response curves) the literature frequently reports and uses concentration units, rather than absolute dose amounts, as the independent variable in these relations. There are both practical and theoretical reasons for using concentration. Clearly, an experiment *in vitro*, e.g., a muscle bath study, would use the amounts of drug that are required in the solution volume containing the tissue. Accordingly, concentrations in units of mg/ml or μg/ml should be used to compare effects and obtain equieffective data. In many systems studied in animals, the volume can only be estimated since it is often not well defined. Commonly we use blood or plasma volume, but intra- or extracellular water might be used — or even total body water. When pharmacokinetic information is adequate to do so, it is preferable to express concentrations in one of these ways when extracting information on equal effects. In whole animal studies, as in analgesic testing, the *apparent volume of distribution* has been used to convert drug doses (amounts) into plasma concentrations; in other studies the doses are expressed in terms of animal body mass, using units such as mg/kg or μg/kg, etc.

Besides these practical reasons there are also other reasons based on theory for using concentrations instead of dose amounts. For example, the law of mass action is usually used as a model of the binding of drugs and chemicals to cellular receptors. This law relates the rate of reaction to the product of the *concentrations* of the reactants (drug and receptor); therefore, studies of the intimate actions of drugs and chemicals require the precision afforded by units of concentration or some other measure used to normalize. Experiments with radioligands often use receptor concentration expressed as pmol per gram of tissue and bound concentrations expressed as fmol per mg of protein. The level of study provides some guidance as to the appropriate ways of expressing concentrations and other dose-related metrics when two or more agents are being studied in a combination experiment. In many descriptions the literature uses the word "dose" (e.g., equieffective dose) in this broader context which includes actual or estimated concentrations or amounts per kg of body weight, per cell, per mg of protein, etc. All of these are used in this book, although some formulas will use notations that distinguish amounts from concentrations. It is therefore necessary to understand the context of these descriptions and formulas.

2.3   Notation

In contrast to the simple symbols x and y that are commonly used in algebra and other mathematical fields, the literature in pharmacology and toxicology usually uses notation that is more suggestive of the meanings of the terms. For example, C is often used for a concentration, V for volume, D for dose, and E for effect. Modifiers with subscripts are frequently used, such as E_{max} for the system maximum effect and E_{maxA} and E_{maxB} for the maximum effects of drugs A and B, respectively. In brief descriptions, that is, in literature sources containing only a few equations, it matters little whether a straight line is described by $y = a + bx$ (as in algebra) or $E = a + b \,(\log C)$, in pharmacological discussions of the effect (E) of some concentration (C) of a drug. However, when one has to incorporate large chunks of mathematical or statistical theory into some dose-effect analysis, e.g., the equations of weighted linear regression, it is convenient to use notations closer to the mathematical field.

In this book, context has guided the choice of symbols to denote pharmacologic quantities. For example, the notation, $ED50$ is so deeply rooted in the pharmacologic description of quantal experiments (as the dose that is effective in 50% of the subjects) that we shall use that term in descriptions even when it is denoted by some other symbol in an equation. In such cases, it will be made clear that the symbol used, for example A, denotes the $ED50$ of drug A. The term "EC50" is also used in pharmacology, denoting the concentration of the drug that gives an effect that is half maximal in graded dose-effect relations, but this usage is less well established. In this book, the notation A_{50} is most often used for that concentration and D_{50} for the corresponding dose as a mole, milligram, or microgram quantity. For example, in Figure 2.1, the A_{50} is 1.56×10^{-6} M for methoxamine HCl.

2.4   Logarithmic transformation

Dose-effect data that exhibit the hyperbolic shape shown in
Figure 2.2a take on a different appearance if the effect is plotted
against the logarithm of the dose as shown in Figure 2.2b. Logarithms
are usually taken to the base ten in such a plot. The transformed
plot is sigmoidal or S-shaped, yet it conveys the same kind of information. If there are sufficient data points in the mid range, (say
between 20 and 80% of the maximum effect) this subset of points
displays a nearly linear trend as shown. In graded dose-effect data,
plotted as effect against log(dose) or log(concentration), this subset
of points is often used to get the drug's A_{50} value. This is accomplished
by the use of a linear equation that best describes the subset of points.
When this equation is derived, as described below, it is used to
calculate the log A_{50} (or log D_{50}) from the equation of the line and
thereby yields the A_{50} as the antilog. This is a quite common way of
obtaining the A_{50} values for drugs that are to be studied in combination and is therefore central to our goal. If some other level of
effect is used the logarithm of its concentration can also be calculated
from the derived linear equation. When the original concentration
unit is transformed by a logarithmic transformation the mean value
of this logarithmic concentration will subsequently be transformed
back to the original unit, thereby yielding the geometric mean concentration. The logarithmic transformation, however, is assumed to
normalize the original measurements of concentration and, thus, the
reversed mean is an estimate of the median in the original concentration unit. Accordingly, the A_{50} found after a regression analysis
that gives log (A_{50}) is termed a *median effective dose*. This topic is
further discussed in the appendix to this chapter.

2.5   Linear regression

As previously mentioned, the relation between the effect of a drug or
chemical and the dose is often transformed to a relation between the
effect and the logarithm of the dose. We denote the effect by y and the
logarithm of the dose (or concentration) by x. The use of the logarithm
produces a plot in Cartesian coordinates that often displays linearity
over some range of x-y values. We now consider how such data produce
an equation for this line. The model, known as the linear regression
model, assumes that there is some true linear relation between the

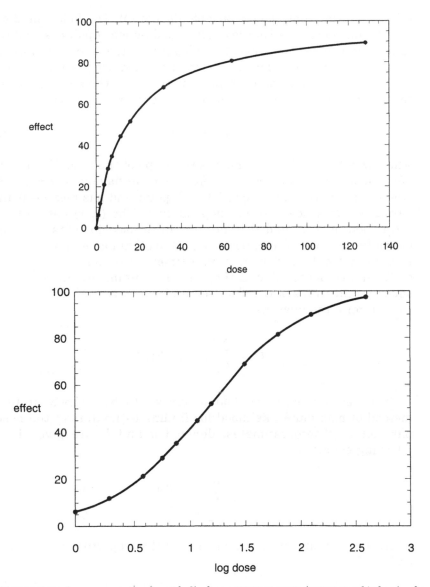

Figure 2.2. A representative hyperbolic dose-response curve (upper graph) that is often used to model pharmacological data. These curves are frequently needed over extensive dose ranges and, therefore, may not clearly accommodate the range of doses and larger effects. Lower graph: Illustration of a transformation of the abscissa to the logarithm of the dose, thereby accommodating a larger dose range and providing a better indication of the maximum effect. The logarithmic transformation results in an S-shaped curve that is approximately linear in the mid-range.

effect y and the controlled x variable (log(dose)). The following discussion, though here aimed at the analysis of dose-effect pairs, is applicable to numerous other situations in which x-y data are to be represented by a straight line relation. The x values which are discrete, x_1, x_2, ... x_i, ... x_N, in our application represent the logarithms of the N doses tested and are assumed to be error free. The mathematical model is

$$y = \alpha + \beta x \qquad (2.1)$$

where α is the y-intercept and β is the slope of the line. The observed effect at any x_i is denoted by y_i. At any x_i we have $y_i = \alpha + \beta x_i + \varepsilon_i$, where ε_i is the random error of the ith point and has mean = 0 and a variance = σ^2 which does not depend on x. The (x, y) data allow an estimation of α, β, and σ^2. The procedure used for obtaining these estimates uses the N data points (x_i, y_i) to obtain an estimated regression line $y = a + bx$. Thus a is an estimate of α and b is an estimate of β. This estimated line is the one that minimizes the sum of the squared differences of the observed and estimated values of y_i. Thus, we minimize the quantity

$$Q = \sum_{i=1}^{N} (y_i - a - bx_i)^2. \qquad (2.2)$$

This least squares method is known to be equivalent to the method of maximum likelihood for finding estimators of the needed parameters. These estimates, denoted a and b, are given by the following equation:

$$b = \frac{\sum x_i y_i - N\bar{x}\bar{y}}{\sum x_i^2 - N\bar{x}^2} \qquad (2.3)$$

where $\bar{x}$ and $\bar{y}$ are the sample means of the respective x and y values and

$$a = \bar{y} - b\bar{x}. \qquad (2.4)$$

Equation 2.4 shows that the estimated regression line passes through the point having the mean x, mean y as coordinates. The residual sum of squares, Q, when divided by $(N - 2)$, is an unbiased estimator of σ^2 and is usually denoted s^2:

$$s^2 = Q/(N-2) \qquad (2.5)$$

The square root of the above, s, is known as the *standard error of estimate*. With a and b determined, the regression line is represented by the equation $Y = a + bx$. In order to distinguish between the y-value of the line and the y-value of a data point, we have used the notation Y for the line value. It represents the mean effect corresponding to $x = \log(\text{dose})$. Since a, b and Y are estimated quantities, each has a variance. These are given by the following equations:

$$V(Y) = s^2\left[\frac{1}{N} + \frac{(x-\bar{x})^2}{\sum(x_i-\bar{x})^2}\right] \qquad (2.6)$$

$$V(a) = s^2\left[\frac{1}{N} + \frac{\bar{x}^2}{\sum(x_i-\bar{x})^2}\right] \qquad (2.7)$$

$$V(b) = \frac{s^2}{\sum(x_i-\bar{x})^2}. \qquad (2.8)$$

It is convenient to represent the denominator, $\sum(x_i-\bar{x})^2$, by the symbol S_{xx}.

From Equation 2.6 it is seen that $V(\bar{y}) = s^2/N$. Most important for our purpose is the variance of the x value that is predicted from the regression line for a given value of Y. For example, Y will be some specified effect level, such as 50% of the maximum, and the corresponding x-value, denoted here by x', is computed from $x' = (Y - a)/b$ with (approximate) variance given by

$$V(x') = \frac{s^2}{b^2}\left[\frac{1}{N} + \frac{(x'-\bar{x})^2}{S_{xx}}\right]. \qquad (2.9)$$

When confidence limits are desired, they are computed from the standard error (SE), the latter computed as the square root of the variance. The half width of the confidence interval is the product, $t(SE)$, where t is a value from Student's distribution for the desired significance level (e.g., $p < 0.05$) and t is based on $(N-2)$ degrees of freedom. Confidence limits computed this way are the true values

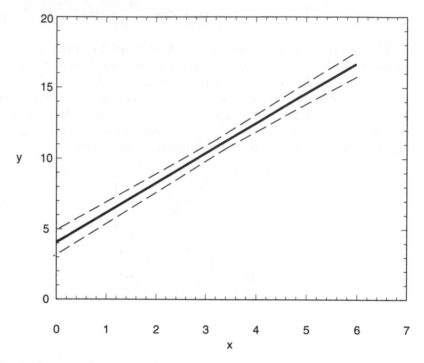

Figure 2.3. Regression line with upper and lower 95% confidence limits (broken lines). The confidence limits are symmetric above and below the line and are minimum at the mean x (in this case $x = 3$).

for the Ys and are symmetric above and below the regression line (Figure 2.3). These confidence bands are hyperbolas (Busby and Tallarida, 1981). It is seen that the confidence limits are a minimum at $\bar{x}$ and widen as the x-values move from the mean. It is noteworthy that the confidence limits of x', computed as $x' \pm tSE(x')$ from Equation 2.9, are also symmetric about x'. But these are approximate confidence limits of x' since the bands are hyperbolas with symmetry in the vertical direction. This approximation is usually acceptable when applied to values of $x' = \log(A_{50})$ used in pharmacological and certain other biological applications. The corresponding A_{50} values, however, would not have symmetric confidence limits since these are obtained as antilogs.

In applications where true confidence limits of x' are needed, these may be computed from the formula below which is equivalent to that given by Bliss (1967, p. 439; in the Bliss formula, the symbol C is used and is related to g by $C - 1 = g/(1 - g)$):

$$x' + \frac{g}{1-g}(x' - \bar{x}) \pm \frac{ts}{b(1-g)}\left[\frac{1-g}{N} + \frac{(x'-\bar{x})^2}{S_{xx}}\right]^{1/2} \qquad (2.10)$$

where

$$g = \frac{t^2 V(b)}{b^2} = \frac{t^2 s^2}{b^2 S_{xx}}. \qquad (2.11)$$

There are many other topics in linear regression that should be included in a more complete discussion, and some of these are covered in the next chapter. Our current objective, however, is to demonstrate the use of linear regression in obtaining concentrations, such as A_{50} or (D_{50}), for a drug in order to have these and their variance estimates that will be used in drug interaction studies. The material presented thus far in this chapter is sufficient for this purpose; the following section illustrates the regression computation.

Determination of D_{50} and its variance from linear regression: example

Studies of the analgesic action of morphine sulfate were conducted in rats in an experiment in which cold water was used as the nociceptive stimulus and the analgesic effect was computed from tail flick latency. This choice of metric produces a continuous measure of analgesia (antinociception) that spans the range 0–100%. Three animals were tested at each dose and produced the data that are given in Table 2.2. A subset of these plotted points, those that exclude doses less than 4.0 mg/kg and greater than 16.0 mg/kg, display a linear trend when the effect is plotted against log(dose) as shown in Figure 2.4. This subset of 5 doses, each tested in 3 animals, was used in a linear regression analysis from which the D_{50}, its variance, and other quantities were calculated. The pertinent calculations are given at the bottom of the table. (The values were modified slightly in order to provide a comprehensive example that illustrates the calculation.)

From the calculated values given in Table 2.2, it follows that the equation of the line is $Y = 108.3x - 47.04$, from which the effect, $Y = 50$, yields $x = \log D_{50} = 0.8960$ and $D_{50} = 7.870$. The variance of log (D_{50}), calculated from Equation 2.9, is $V(\log D_{50}) = (3.163^2/108.3^2) [1/15 + (0.8960 - 0.9028)^2/0.6796] = 0.00005696$ and thus, $SE = 0.007547$. Multiplication of this SE by $t = 2.160$ (95% and d.f.= 13) gives 0.01630,

Table 2.2. Dose-Effect Data for Morphine Sulfate in Rat Cold-Water Test

Dose	Log(dose)	Effect
	x	y
2.00	0.301	4.00
2.00	0.301	9.00
2.00	0.301	16.0
4.00	0.602	16.0
4.00	0.602	18.0
4.00	0.602	21.0
5.65	0.752	32.0
5.65	0.752	36.0
5.65	0.752	39.0
8.00	0.903	45.0
8.00	0.903	51.0
8.00	0.903	52.0
11.3	1.05	62.0
11.3	1.05	66.0
11.3	1.05	68.0
16.0	1.20	82.0
16.0	1.20	85.0
16.0	1.20	88.0
32.0	1.50	99.0
32.0	1.50	100
32.0	1.50	100

Summary of regression calculations

$\Sigma x = 13.54$, $\Sigma y = 761$, $N = 15$, $\bar{x} = 0.9028$, $\bar{y} = 50.73$

$\Sigma x^2 = 12.91$, $\Sigma xy = 760.6$, $b = 108.3$, $a = -47.04$, $Q = 130.1$

$s = 3.163$, $S_{xx} = 0.6796$, $g = 0.00586$, $V(b) = 14.72$, $t = 2.160$

Data supplied by M.W. Adler from a preliminary study that was subsequently used in a larger investigation (Chen et al., 1996).

a value added and subtracted from 0.8960 to give the confidence interval (0.8797 to 0.9123). Because g is so small, this confidence interval is virtually identical to the true value computed from Equation 2.11. This is an interval for log (D_{50}); antilogs give the 95% confidence interval of the D_{50}: 7.580 to 8.171 mg/kg.

In many applications one needs the standard error of D_{50}. The results of regression analysis, which are usually on log(dose) as in this

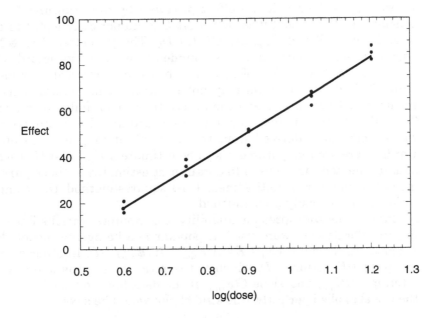

Figure 2.4. Analgesia in rats plotted against log(dose) of morphine sulfate (mg/kg, s.c.). The nociceptive stimulus was cold water; the effect, antinociception, was determined from tail flick latency as described by Chen et al., 1996.

example, give the *SE* of this logarithm. In such cases an approximation that is often acceptable (see appendix) is given below:

$$SE(D_{50}) = 2.30 \times D_{50} \times SE(\log D_{50}). \qquad (2.12)$$

In the current example this standard error is $2.30 \times 7.870 \times 0.007547 = 0.1366$.

2.6   Nonlinear models

The previous example used the logarithm of the dose and the subset of data points showing a somewhat linear trend. When all the points are used and the effect (E) is plotted against the dose (D), rather than its logarithm, the points are often modeled as a hyperbola

$$E = E_{max}D/(D + C) \qquad (2.13)$$

where E_{max} is the maximum effect produced by the drug and C is a constant. In this model it is seen that C is numerically equal to the dose that gives $E = 1/2\ E_{max}$, i.e., C is the D_{50}. The graph (see Figure 2.5) passes through the origin and is bounded from above in accord with the notion that the effect of any drug has some practical maximum value. This drug maximum may not be attained in realistic experiments since large doses may be impractical for any number of reasons. Thus, the maximum effect may have to be estimated from analysis of the smooth curve derived from the available data points. In other words, there are two parameters to be estimated: E_{max} and C. A least squares method can be used to obtain best estimates of these parameters, but, in contrast to the linear least squares method, this computation is not so easily accomplished.

Prior to the widespread availability of computers, various linearizing transformations were used, a popular one being the model that reciprocates the data, i.e., $1/E = 1/E_{max} + (C/E_{max})\ 1/D$. In other words, one plots $1/E$ against $1/D$, which is theoretically a straight line with intercept, $1/E_{max}$, and slope C/E_{max}. If the data had no variability and the model applied perfectly, this kind of plot would be a convenient and

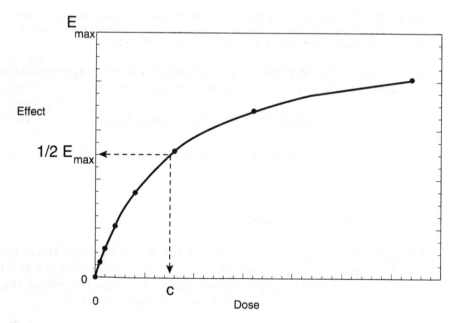

Figure 2.5. In the hyperbolic model, the constant C is the value of the dose (or concentration) that corresponds to an effect level on the curve equal to half the maximum effect.

simple way to determine both C and E_{max}. Because neither of these assumptions is true, the reciprocated points show scatter. It may therefore seem reasonable to use the linear least squares method (regression) to fit the points to a line derived this way, and, indeed, this has been done in many pharmacologic and biochemical analyses. The results are often incorrect because the $1/E$ values display unequal variances over the range of values, a phenomenon that is not in accord with the underlying regression theory. This may be practically appreciated when one considers the small effects produced by small doses. Even slight errors in E produce extreme variations in the reciprocals. At the upper end, near the maximum, there is a huge variation in dose for any effect as the curve "flattens," and this large variability is reflected in the reciprocated dose values. A possible remedy is to employ weights that equalize the variance; a practical approach is to use a nonlinear curve fitting program on the actual D, E data pairs. (See Chapter 11.)

If properly fitted hyperbolas are obtained for two full agonists (thus, each attains the same maximum), for example, $E = E_{max} D/(D + C_1)$ and $E = E_{max}D/(D + C_2)$, the equieffective doses have the relative potency $R = C_1/C_2$, a constant equal to the ratio of their respective D_{50} values. In other words the relative potency is a constant, independent of the effect level in this case, a fact that greatly simplifies analysis of the combined action to be discussed in Chapter 4. Some dose-effect data that are approximately described by a hyperbola (Equation 2.13) are sometimes better modeled from

$$E = \frac{E_{max}D^p}{D^p + C^p} \qquad (2.14)$$

where p has a value other than one. For example, the methoxamine data of Table 2.1 was modeled with the curve-fitting parameter, $p = 1.4$. A discussion of this procedure is given in Chapter 11.

Appendix

The expected value (mean value) of the random variable x is here denoted by $E(x)$ and its variance by σ^2. We are concerned in our applications with logarithms of some specified dose, e.g, log D_{50}, the variance, Var (log D_{50}), and the relation of these to D_{50} and $Var(D_{50})$. The mean value of log (D_{50}) and its variance are obtained from linear regression of effect on log(dose) and therefore one cannot get the true standard error of the D_{50}. An approximation is obtained if the following apply:

If

(i) $$\mu = E\{\log D_{50}\}$$

(ii) $$\sigma^2 = Var\{\log D_{50}\}$$

and

(iii)   log $\{D_{50}\}$ is normally distributed,

then

$$E\{D_{50}\} = e^{(\ln 10)\mu + \frac{1}{2}(\ln 10)^2\sigma^2}$$
$$= 10^{\mu}e^{\frac{1}{2}(\ln 10)^2\sigma^2}$$

(A2.1)

and

$$Var\{D_{50}\} = 10^{2\mu}e^{(\ln 10)^2\sigma^2}[e^{(\ln 10)^2\sigma^2} - 1].$$ (A2.2)

Equation A2.1 points out that the mean D_{50} is not the antilog of log D_{50}.

What one gets from the antilog is the geometric mean which, in the effectively normalized transformation, is an estimate of the median D_{50}. In pharmacologic work this median D_{50}, rather than the true mean (expected value), is the quantity usually used and quoted.

For sufficiently small σ^2 the above bracketed term in Equation A2.2 $\approx (\ln 10)^2 \sigma^2$; thus

$$Var\{D_{50}\} \approx [E\{D_{50}\}]^2 (2.30)^2 \sigma^2,$$

from which the more familiar standard error formula (Finney, 1971, p.36) follows by taking square roots:

$$SE\{D_{50}\} \approx 2.30 E\{D_{50}\} SE\{\log D_{50}\} \qquad (A2.3)$$

which is also Equation 2.12. Bliss (1967, p.128) gives a slightly different (but equivalent form) of Equation A2.1:

$$E\{D_{50}\} = 10^{\left(\mu + \frac{1}{2}\ln 10 \sigma^2\right)}$$

which he writes as the antilog $(\log D_{50} + 1.1513\, s^2)$, where s^2 denotes the sample variance. A *heuristic* approach using differentials to approximate standard errors on original and logarithmic scales leads to Equation 2.12 more directly. In familiar symbols,

if $$y = \log_{10} x \approx (\ln x)/2.30$$

$$dy \approx (1/2.30)\, dx/x;$$

hence,

$$dx \approx (2.30)\, x\, dy$$

In words, the error in D_{50} is approximately $2.30 \times D_{50} \times$ error of $\log (D_{50})$.

CHAPTER 2

References

Ariens, E.J. *Molecular Pharmacology*, V. 1, Academic Press, New York, 1964.

Bliss, C.I. *Statistics in Biology*, V. 1. McGraw-Hill, New York, 1967.

Busby, R.C. and Tallarida, R.J. On the analysis of straight-line data in pharmacology and biochemistry. *J. Theor. Biol.* 93:867–879, 1981.

Chen, X.H., Liu-Chen, L.Y., Tallarida, R.J., Geller, E.B., de Riel, J.K., and Adler, M.W. Use of a mu-antisense oligodeoxynucleotide as a mu-opioid receptor noncompetitive antagonist in vivo. *Neurochem. Res.* 21:1363–68, 1996.

Finney, D.J. *Probit Analysis*, 3rd ed. Cambridge, 1971.

Goldstein, A., Aronow, L., and Kalman, S.M. *Principles of Drug Action*, 2nd ed. Wiley, New York, 1974.

Kenakin, T.P. *Pharmacologic Analysis of Drug-Receptor Interaction*. 3rd ed. Lippincott Williams and Wilkins, Philadelphia, 1997.

Lauffenburger, D.A. and Linderman, J.J. *Receptors*. Oxford University Press, Oxford, 1993.

Pizziketti, R.J., Pressman, N.S., Geller, E.B., Cowan, A., and Adler, M.W. Rat cold water tail-flick: A novel analgesic test that distinguishes opioid agonists from mixed agonist-antagonists. *Eur. J. Pharmacol.* 119:23–29, 1985.

Raffa, R.B., Tallarida, R.J., and Gero, A. Determination of the stimulus-response relation for three alpha-adrenergic agonists on rabbit aorta. *Arch. Int. Pharmacodyn. Ther.* 241: 197–207, 1979.

Tallarida, R.J. and Jacob, L.S. *The Dose-Response Relation in Pharmacology*. Springer-Verlag, New York, 1979.

Tallarida, R.J., Raffa, R.B., and McGonigle, P. *Principles in General Pharmacology*. Springer-Verlag, New York, 1988.

Linear Regression:
A Further Discussion

Linear regression was introduced in the previous chapter. We now provide a more detailed discussion of this topic. Our aim is to calculate potency values (such as D_{50}) from regression lines that are modeled on a logarithmic scale, i.e., as effect vs. log dose. These potencies are needed in isobolar combination analysis discussed in the next chapter. Here we will be especially concerned with tests of the parallelism of the regression lines of effect on log dose and the importance of this in combination drug analysis. The concepts and methods presented here will have many other applications also. When it is necessary to distinguish between an observed y-value, y_i, and the corresponding value on the line, the latter will be denoted with a capital letter, Y_i, as we did in the previous chapter. Thus, the regression line is written, $Y = a + bx$, and at any x-value, x_i, we have $Y_i = a + bx_i$. A first objective is to test the hypothesis that the slope β, which is estimated as b, is significantly different from zero. (For log(dose)-effect data this is a test to determine whether the effect is dose dependent.) We shall present two different tests for this purpose. The first uses an analysis of variance (ANOVA).

3.1   ANOVA in linear regression

The N observed values y_i have a mean value that we have denoted $\bar{y}$. The sum of squared differences, $\sum (y_i - \bar{y})^2$, is calculated and is denoted here SS_t

$$SS_t = \sum (y_i - \bar{y})^2 . \tag{3.1}$$

The quantity SS_t is a measure of the overall variability of the y values; it includes a part due to the regression and a part due to the deviations about the line. The part due to regression is denoted SS_{reg} and is given by

$$SS_{reg} = \sum (Y_i - \bar{y})^2. \tag{3.2}$$

SS_{reg} is a measure of the deviation of the y values of the line from the sample mean. The part due to deviation about the line is called the residual sum of squares SS_{res} (denoted Q in Chapter 2) and is given by

$$SS_{res} = \sum (y_i - Y_i)^2. \tag{3.3}$$

These sums of squares are related as follows:

$$SS_t = SS_{reg} + SS_{res}. \tag{3.4}$$

SS_t has degrees of freedom $= N - 1$, whereas that due to regression has 1 degree of freedom and that due to SS_{res} has $(N - 2)$ degrees of freedom. Division of each SS by its degrees of freedom gives the mean square (MS). It is common to display these relations in a table such as Table 3.1. It should be noted that MS_{res} is the quantity previously denoted by s^2 in Equation 2.5, i.e., the square of the standard error of estimate. A test of the hypothesis that $\beta = 0$ (slope $= 0$) is made from the F-distribution (Table A.9) by first calculating the ratio

$$F = MS_{reg} / MS_{res} \tag{3.5}$$

and comparing it with the critical F for degrees of freedom 1 (across) and $N - 2$ (down) at the level of significance desired (e.g., $p < 0.05$). If the calculated value exceeds the tabular value of F then β is significantly different from 0. The calculated sum of squares terms allow a calculation

Table 3.1. ANOVA Summary in Simple Linear Regression

Source of Variation	Sum of Squares (SS)	Degrees of Freedom (DF)	Mean Square (MS)
Total	SS_t	$N - 1$	$MS_{reg} = SS_{reg} / 1$
Regression	SS_{reg}	1	$MS_{res} = SS_{res} / (N - 2)$
Residual	SS_{res}	$N - 2$	$F = MS_{reg} / MS_{res}$

of the *coefficient of determination*, denoted r^2, and given by the following equation:

$$r^2 = SS_{reg} / SS_t. \qquad (3.6)$$

This value is an indicator of the proportion of the total variation that is accounted for by the regression line. (Its square root, r, is the correlation coefficient used in correlation analysis.) A value of r^2 near 1 indicates that the variation in the y-values is mainly due to regression while a value near zero indicates that this variation is not well accounted for by the regression line.

> **Example**. The data used in Table 2.2 were fitted to a line given by the equation, $Y = 108.307 \, x - 47.046$. A summary of the analysis of variance is shown in Table 3.2. The calculated $F = 796.527$, whereas the critical value, based on degrees of freedom 1 and 13 for $p < 0.05$ (95% level), is 4.67, and for $p < 0.01$ (99% level) it is 9.07. Because the calculated F greatly exceeds the tabular 9.07, this result indicates that the slope is significantly different from zero, and well beyond the 99% level, that is, the effect is clearly dose dependent. The coefficient of determination, r^2, is 0.984 so scatter about the line is rather small. Stated differently, 98.4% of the variation in effect is due to regression. The detailed regression calculations are summarized in Table 2.2 and its accompanying text.

The t-Test in Linear Regression. The hypothesis tested with the F-statistic can also be tested with the t-distribution. This calculation uses the estimated slope b and its variance $V(b)$ to calculate t as follows:

$$t = b/\{V(b)\}^{1/2}. \qquad (3.7)$$

The value calculated from the above is compared to the critical t, for $N - 2$ degrees of freedom at the significance level desired, e.g., 95%.

Table 3.2. ANOVA for Linear Regression of Analgesia on Log (Morphine Sulfate)

Source of Variation	Sum of Squares (SS)	Degrees of Freedom (DF)	Mean Square (MS)
Total	8100.934	14	
Regression	7970.846	1	7970.846
Residual	130.088	13	10.007
			$F = 796.527$

See Table 2.2.

(See Table A.6). If the calculated t exceeds the critical value from the table, we reject the hypothesis that the slope is zero. In other words, the slope is significantly different from 0. In the above example the calculated $t = 28.223$ and the tabular value (for 95% and d.f. = 13) is 2.160; for 99% the tabular value is 3.012. Therefore, in this example, the result is highly significant. Of course, the same conclusion was reached with the calculation of F; in fact, it may be noted that the calculated t and F values are related as $t^2 = F$ in these tests.

3.2   Parallel line analysis

Sometimes the chemical properties or known mechanisms of two different drugs suggest that their regression lines, for the same effect on log(dose), should be parallel. Statistical methods exist for testing whether two regression lines are parallel.

Parallel regression lines of effect on log(dose) mean that the relative potency of the compounds is constant over the range of effects. (When the difference, $\log(A) - \log(B)$, is constant, it follows that $R = A/B$ is constant.) Considerable attention has been given to such cases in the pharmacological literature so that some discussion here is appropriate. When the regression line is *probit* against log(dose), discussed later in Chapter 6 on quantal responses, the slope of the line is $1/\sigma$, the reciprocal of the standard deviation of log($ED50$). Thus, if the standard deviations for the two different compounds are equal, it follows that their probit regression lines are parallel. Besides this very important property in probit analysis, the use of parallel regression lines is important enough to include in this discussion of simple linear regression.

Test for parallelism

Two regression lines, lines (1) and (2), with respective estimated slopes b_1 and b_2, will have been determined along with the quantities expressed in an analysis of variance of each. The numbers of points in the regressions are N_1 and N_2, respectively. The hypothesis to be tested is that *the difference, $b_1 - b_2 = 0$*, and the test utilizes the t-distribution. The residual sum of squares values from each line are used in a calculation of a *pooled standard error of estimate, s*, from the relation

$$s^2 = \frac{SS_{res(1)} + SS_{res(2)}}{(N_1 - 2) + (N_2 - 2)}. \tag{3.8}$$

In pooling for this application it is assumed that the values of s^2 of each line are equal. Next, the value of t is calculated and compared to the critical t for degrees of freedom, d.f. $= N_1 + N_2 - 4$ at the specified level of significance, e.g., $p < 0.05$, according to

$$t = \frac{|b_1 - b_2|}{s(1/S_{xx(1)} + 1/S_{xx(2)})^{1/2}} . \qquad (3.9)$$

If the t calculated from Equation 3.9 exceeds the critical value (Table A.6) then we reject the hypothesis of equality of slopes; otherwise, we accept the hypothesis that the difference in slopes is not significant. The following example illustrates these computations.

Example. *Cocaine and Buprenorphine.* The psychomotor stimulating effects of cocaine are well known and have prompted studies aimed at quantitating these effects as a function of dose. The data below, from the laboratory of S.G. Holtzman (Emory University), compared rotational behavior in the rat induced by graded doses of cocaine with the same behavior induced by buprenorphine, a partial *mu*-opioid thought to enhance some of the behavioral and neurochemical actions of cocaine (Kimmel et al., 1997). The effect metric is based on rotational behavior in animals with surgically induced unilateral nigral lesions that subsequently received the drug treatments. Figure 3.1 shows the regression lines. The data are given in Table 3.3 and show the number of turns (over control) in a specified time interval that were observed at each

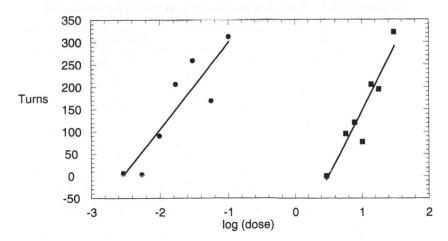

Figure 3.1. Regression of effect on log dose for cocaine (right curve) and buprenorphine (left curve). The effect is the increase in turns over control values.

dose (mg/kg) for each drug and the results of the regression analysis needed to compare the slopes. It is notable that the estimated slopes, 302.80 and 201.92, differ, but it is also evident that the large standard errors $(SE(b))$ suggest that a statistical test is needed. Application of Equation 3.8 to the regression outputs gives $s^2 = (7953.65 + 16857.17)/10 = 2481.08$, so that $s = 49.81$, while $1/S_{xx(1)} + 1/S_{xx(2)} = 2.094$. Use of these values in Equation 3.9 yields $t = (302.80 - 201.92)/[(49.81)(2.094)^{1/2}] = 1.40$, a value whose magnitude does not exceed the critical value of $t_{10, 0.05} = 2.228$ given in Table A.6. Because the slopes could not be shown to differ significantly, we proceed to estimate a common slope as discussed in the next section.

3.3 The common slope and relative potency

The regression line, $Y = a + bx$, passes through the point $(\bar{x}, \bar{y})$, and, therefore, its equation may be written in the form $Y = \bar{y} + b(x - \bar{x})$. This form is convenient in this section in which we discuss parallel regression lines. The object is to find the common slope b_c from two lines whose estimated slopes are b_1 and b_2. In our application these will be the regression lines of two different drugs, but the method may be used whenever there is an indication for constraining lines to parallel.

Table 3.3. Comparing Slopes of Two Regression Lines: Cocaine and Buprenorphine in the Production of Rotation in the Nigrally-Lesioned Rat

Cocaine			Buprenorphine		
Dose	Log(dose)	Turns	Dose	Log(dose)	Turns
3.00	0.477	0	0.003	−2.522	5
5.60	0.748	97	0.0056	−2.252	2
7.50	0.875	121	0.010	−2.000	90
10.0	1.000	78	0.017	−1.770	207
13.3	1.123	208	0.030	−1.523	260
17.5	1.243	198	0.056	−1.252	170
30.0	1.477	326	0.100	−1.000	314

$a = -153.48; b = 302.80; SE(b) = 49.32$ $a = 505.09; b = 201.92; SE(b) = 43.60$

$N = 7; S_{xx} = 0.654; SS_{res} = 7937; r^2 = 0.88$ $N = 7; S_{xx} = 1.77; SS_{res} = 16852; r^2 = 0.81$

$\bar{x} = 0.9919; \bar{y} = 146.86$ $\bar{x} = -1.760; \bar{y} = 149.71$

Doses are in units of mg/kg; cocaine was administered i.p. and buprenorphine s.c.

The individual regression lines for drugs 1 and 2 are given by

$$Y = \bar{y}_{(1)} + b_1(x - \bar{x}_{(1)})$$

and

$$Y = \bar{y}_{(2)} + b_2(x - \bar{x}_{(2)}).$$

The common slope b_c is determined from the N_1 points of drug 1 and the N_2 points of drug 2 according to

$$b_c = [S_{xy(1)} + S_{xy(2)}] / [S_{xx(1)} + S_{xx(2)}] \qquad (3.10)$$

where $S_{xy} = \Sigma (x_i - \bar{x}) (y_i - \bar{y})$, S_{xx} is defined as previously, and the subscripted parentheses indicate summation over the respective data sets. (The common slope was derived as the weighted mean of the individual regression slopes, using as weights the reciprocal of $V(b)$ and a pooled estimate of s^2, given below as Equation 3.13.) The cross term sums in the above may be computed more conveniently from the relation for each line:

$$\sum(x_i - \bar{x})(y_i - \bar{y}) = \sum x_i y_i - N\bar{x}\bar{y} \qquad (3.11)$$

The parallel regression lines are given by

$$Y = \bar{y}_{(1)} + b_c(x - \bar{x}_{(1)})$$
$$Y = \bar{y}_{(2)} + b_c(x - \bar{x}_{(2)}).$$

The common slope allows an estimation of the horizontal distance M between lines 1 and 2 (Figure 3.2). M is given by

$$M = \bar{x}_{(1)} - \bar{x}_{(2)} - (\bar{y}_{(1)} - \bar{y}_{(2)})/b_c. \qquad (3.12)$$

In our application x is the logarithm of dose (or concentration), so the quantity M is the logarithm of the relative potency R; thus $R = 10^M$.

We now want to get confidence limits for M and, thus, for the relative potency R. For this purpose we need the sum of squares of residuals from each regression line in order to get a pooled estimate of the error variance s_p^2 which is given by

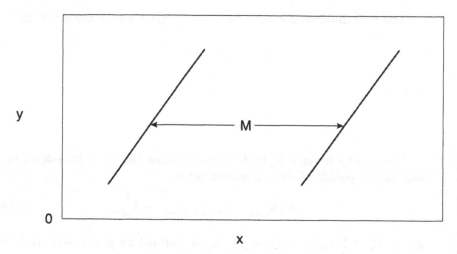

Figure 3.2. Horizontal distance M between parallel regression lines. When the x-axis is log dose the value of M is the logarithm of the relative potency.

$$s_p^2 = [SS_{res(1)} + SS_{res(2)}]/(N_1 + N_2 - 3). \qquad (3.13)^*$$

This, in turn, is used in calculating the variance of the common slope,

$$V(b_c) = s_p^2/(S_{xx(1)} + S_{xx(2)}) \qquad (3.14)$$

and from these, $V(M)$ follows as

$$V(M) = (1/b_c^2)[s_p^2/N_1 + s_p^2/N_2 + (\bar{x}_{(1)} - \bar{x}_{(2)} - M)^2 V(b_c)]. \quad (3.15)$$

The above expression for $V(M)$ is an approximation and therefore confidence limits based on it, given by $M \pm t\,[V(M)]^{1/2}$, are symmetric (and also approximate). In this application t has degrees of freedom = $N_1 + N_2 - 3$. With upper (M_u) and lower (M_l) limits on M calculated it is possible to get the confidence limits of R:

$$R_{lower} = 10^{M_l}; \quad R_{upper} = 10^{M_u}. \qquad (3.16)$$

Example. The potency ratio and its confidence limits are to be calculated from the data on cocaine and buprenorphine in Table 3.3 (Tallarida et

---

*Degrees of freedom are now $N_1 + N_2 - 3$; see, for example, Draper and Smith, 2nd ed. 1981, (p. 58, Ex. D).

al., 1997). We begin by getting the common slope. For this we need the sum of cross terms, $\sum (x_i - \bar{x})(y_i - \bar{y})$ for each line. These are most easily computed from Equation 3.11. For cocaine (drug 1) the sum of cross terms is 197.9, and for buprenorphine (drug 2) the value is 358.4. The common slope is

$$b_c = (197.9 + 358.4)/(0.654 + 1.77)$$

$$= 229.5.$$

The parallel regression lines are

$$Y = 146.86 + 229.5 \ (x - 0.9919) \quad \text{(cocaine)}$$

$$Y = 149.7 + 229.5 \ (x + 1.760) \quad \text{(buprenorphine)}.$$

The horizontal distance between them is

$$M = (0.9919 + 1.760) - (146.86 - 149.71)/(229.5)$$

$$= 2.764.$$

The estimated relative potency $R = 10^M = 580.8$.

The following calculations are directed toward getting the confidence limits of R.

For this we need the pooled error variance,

$$s_p^2 = (7937 + 16852)/(11)$$

$$= 2254.5$$

and the slope variance,

$$V(b_c) = 2254/(0.654 + 1.77)$$

$$= 929.9.$$

The variance of M is

$$V(M) = 1/(229.5)^2[2254/7 + 2254/7 + (-0.0121)^2(929.9)]$$

$$= 0.01223 \ ; \text{ thus } SE(M) = 0.1106.$$

The value of t (df $= 11$ and $p = 0.05$) is 2.201 and approximate confidence limits of M are calculated as $M \pm t\ SE(M)$:

$$2.764 \pm (2.201)(0.1106) = 2.764 \pm 0.2434.$$

Thus,

$$M_l = 2.521$$

and

$$M_u = 3.007$$

so the potency ratio R, estimated as 580.8, has 95% confidence limits.

$$R_l = 10^{2.521} = 331.9$$

and

$$R_u = 10^{3.007} = 1016.$$

3.4   Confidence limits of the potency ratio

The confidence limits for R, calculated from the variance formula of Equation 3.15, are often sufficient. The approximation is good if the quantity $g = t^2\ V(b)/b_c^2$ is small, say less than 0.1. In the preceding example $g = 0.086$. When this condition is not met, or when greater precision is needed, the exact confidence limits for M are first obtained from the following:

$$[\bar{x}_{(1)} - \bar{x}_{(2)}] + [\{M - \bar{x}_{(1)} + \bar{x}_{(2)}\}/(1-g)]$$
$$\pm\{tL/[b_c(1-g)]\} \tag{3.17}$$

where L is given by

$$L = \{[M - \bar{x}_{(1)} + \bar{x}_{(2)}]^2 V(b_c) + (1-g)[V(\bar{y}_{(1)}) + V(\bar{y}_{(2)})]\}^{1/2}. \tag{3.18}$$

These limits are then used in Equation 3.16 to get the limits of the potency ratio.

It should be noted that if g can be neglected, these confidence limits reduce to

$$M \pm t\{V(M)\}^{1/2}. \tag{3.19}$$

3.5   Weighted least square regression

When simple regression analysis is carried out, it is assumed that the error variance of ε_i is constant and equal to σ^2. When these variances are unequal, say σ_i^2, a weighting term w_i is used and chosen proportional to $1/\sigma_i^2$, say $w_i = \sigma^2/\sigma_i^2$. This has the effect of assigning less weight to observations y_i that have a large variance and more weight to those observations with less variance. (This idea is especially important in discussions of quantal dose-effect data presented in a later chapter in addition to sufficient importance for discussion here also.) In the special case that all $w_i = 1$, the simple regression model is obtained. In weighted linear regression, the computations are made from the formulas given in the appendix to this chapter.

CHAPTER 3

Appendix 3

The linear regression model, $Y = \alpha x + \beta$, estimated as $Y = a + bx$ in weighted linear regression, calculates values from the following formulas:

$$\bar{x} = \frac{\sum w_i x_i}{\sum w_i}; \; \bar{y} = \frac{\sum w_i y_i}{\sum w_i} \tag{A3.1}$$

$$b = \frac{\sum w_i x_i y_i - \bar{x}\bar{y}\sum w_i}{\sum w_i x_i^2 - \bar{x}^2 \sum w_i} \tag{A3.2}$$

$$a = \bar{y} - b\bar{x} \tag{A3.3}$$

$$s^2 = \frac{\sum w_i (Y_i - y_i)^2}{N-2} \tag{A3.4}$$

$$V(b) = \frac{s^2}{\sum w_i (x_i - \bar{x})^2} \tag{A3.5}$$

$$V(a) = s^2 \left[\frac{1}{\sum w_i} + \frac{\bar{x}^2}{\sum w_i (x_i - \bar{x})^2} \right] \tag{A3.6}$$

$$V(Y) = s^2 \left[\frac{1}{\sum w_i} + \frac{(x - \bar{x})^2}{\sum w_i (x_i - \bar{x})^2} \right] \tag{A3.7}$$

$$V(x') \approx \frac{s^2}{b^2} \left[\frac{1}{\sum w_i} + \frac{(x' - \bar{x})^2}{\sum w_i (x_i - \bar{x})^2} \right] \tag{A3.8}$$

CHAPTER 3

References

Draper, N. and Smith, H. *Applied Regression Analysis*, 2nd ed. John Wiley, New York, 1981.

Kimmel, H.L., Tallarida, R.J., and Holtzman, S.G. Synergism between buprenorphine and cocaine on the rotational behavior of the nigrally-lesioned rat. *Psychopharmacology* 133:372–377, 1997.

Tallarida, R.J., Kimmel, H.L., and Holtzman, S.G. Theory and statistics of detecting synergism between two active drugs: Cocaine and buprenorphine. *Psychopharmacology* 133:378–382, 1997.

Calculations for Combination Drug Analysis

In this chapter we illustrate the calculations that permit a distinction between additive and non-additive interactions of drugs. As we saw earlier, dose-effect data of the constituent compounds are needed for this purpose. Specifically we need equieffective doses (or concentrations) A and B of cxompounds A and B, respectively, that produce the *specified effect* and combination doses a of compound A and b of compound B that give this effect when present together. Additive combinations are those that obey Equation 1.3, $a/A + b/B = 1$. The estimates A and B will have been determined from the individual dose-effect data of the compounds, using methods of analysis discussed in the preceding chapters that also yield variances of these estimated quantities. (Methods of getting these from *quantal* data use probit or logit analysis discussed in Chapter 6, but, in either case, the following discussion is applicable.) For graded dose-effect data the values usually are derived from linear regression of effect on log(dose) or from the hyperbolic model of effect vs. dose obtained from nonlinear curve analysis. Whether the data are graded or quantal, the first consideration is to determine how much of each constituent should be used in a combination experiment. How does one design an experiment, i.e., test various dose combinations, and then subsequently analyze the data to distinguish between additive and nonadditive interactions?

4.1 Experimental designs

Several different experimental designs have been used for this purpose. One approach was illustrated in the method of analysis used in the alcohol-chloral hydrate experiments discussed in Chapter 1. In that study, the investigators constructed the "line of additivity" defined by the individual drugs' *ED50* values (quantal data), and then they obtained the values of doses a and b that gave the 50% effect as a combination. To accomplish that, the dose of one of the drugs (drug B) was fixed at the value b, and the experiment consisted of adding increasing amounts of drug A so the 50% effect could be determined. This amount of drug A is, therefore, an estimated quantity which we shall here denote a_{mix} (for mixture); its variance is denoted $V(a_{mix})$. The plotted point (a, b) therefore has error bars in one direction (the "a-axis"). It is necessary to compare this with the corresponding additive quantity a_{add} calculated from the line of additivity ($a/A + b/B = 1$). Thus a_{add} is estimated from this equation: $a_{add} = A - b(A/B)$. But this too has a variance, $V(a_{add})$. This variance may not be easy to calculate for several reasons. First, there is the problem of dealing with the ratio, $A/B = R$, of quantities that contain error. There is no simple way to get the variance of R precisely (although approximate methods exist); further, we need to get additional quantities (such as the covariance) that are expressed in the formula for $V(a_{add})$,

$$V(a_{add}) = V(A) + b^2 V(R) - 2 b \ cov(A, R).$$

Besides the complexity seen in the above formula, there is the practical reality that A and B often have large variances and the variance of $R = A/B$ and the other terms above are magnified. Accordingly, this design may not be useful for practical purposes, a fact seemingly recognized by the investigators in the alcohol-chloral hydrate study who also used an alternate experimental design in which the components were administered in a *fixed-ratio combination*. Few details of this kind of analysis were provided by the investigators. The advantages of a fixed-ratio design have been described (Tallarida, 1992; Tallarida et al., 1989, 1997). The following section presents the main ideas and the calculations needed in this approach.

4.2   Fixed-ratio design

In a fixed-ratio design the constituents are administered in amounts that keep the proportions of each constant. This design is desirable for several reasons. A manufactured combination product would certainly contain a constant proportion of the ingredients. Also, in experimental work, this design simplifies the analysis of the data. Finally, it has been found that synergism, when it occurs, is a function of the proportions in the combination; i.e., one proportion may be markedly synergistic while another is simply additive. Analysis of data from this design is now described.

An effect level that is reached by each constituent should be chosen. For two full agonists this level is usually 50% of the maximum effect. The individual effective doses of the constituents (those that produce the specified effect) are then estimated as doses (or concentrations) A and B, along with their variances $V(A)$ and $V(B)$, respectively, as previously described (see Chapter 2). For illustrative purposes, let us say that these are D_{50} doses. These values provide a guide to the quantities of the respective agents that are to be used in a combination. The combination doses are taken to be fractions of each compound's D_{50} such that the fractions add to unity: f and $(1 - f)$. The D_{50} of drug A is denoted A, and that of drug B is denoted B. If A and B were known precisely, then the amounts in an additive combination are $a = fA$ of compound A and $b = (1 - f)B$ of compound B. Amounts chosen in this way are clearly additive for the production of this level of effect since they satisfy the equation, $a/A + b/B = 1$. When these amounts are expressed in common mass units (e.g., mg or μg quantities) the total amount in the mixture is the sum, here denoted, Z_{add}:

$$Z_{add} = fA + (1 - f)B. \tag{4.1}$$

The quantities A and B are not known precisely. Their estimated values from dose-effect analysis are used in determining the fixed ratio combination to be tested; hence, the precise proportions of each are based on these estimates and the choice of fraction f. The proportions are precise: $\rho_A = fA/Z_{add}$ and $\rho_B = (1 - f)B/Z_{add}$. The combination with these proportions is administered as though it were a new, third compound. To simplify this discussion, we refer to this combination as a *third compound*. (It is a mixture and not a compound, in the chemical sense).

The third compound is then administered in varying doses in order to determine the actual amount, denoted Z_{mix}, that is needed to produce the desired effect. This amount is obtained as an estimate from the dose-effect data of the third compound using some appropriate method such as linear regression (or nonlinear curve fitting) along with its variance $V(Z_{mix})$. Thus, the combination data provide Z_{mix} and its variance, and Equation 4.1 gives the calculated total in an additive combination, Z_{add}. A statistical test on these two totals requires the variance of Z_{add}. Whereas the fraction f is assumed to be under precise control of the investigator (and, thus, error free), there is uncertainty in Z_{add} because A and B are uncertain so that this quantity has a variance given by

$$V(Z_{add}) = f^2 V(A) + (1 - f)^2 \, V(B). \qquad (4.2)$$

A statistical test of significance $(Z_{add} - Z_{mix})$ is made from the derived and calculated values. If the difference is not significantly different from zero we conclude that the combination is simply additive. In contrast, a significant difference indicates nonadditivity as follows:

synergism if $\qquad\qquad\qquad Z_{mix} < Z_{add} \qquad\qquad\qquad\qquad$ (4.3)

sub-additivity if $\qquad\qquad\qquad Z_{mix} > Z_{add.} \qquad\qquad\qquad\qquad$ (4.4)

A method for testing the significance of the difference, $Z_{mix} - Z_{add}$, is given in the following section. It should be recalled that the parameter estimates, A, B, their variances and all data from the combination (third compound) are quantities that come from the selection of a particular effect level. There are practical and theoretical reasons for selecting an effect in the mid range, such as 50% of the maximum, but other levels of effect can be used provided all dose-effect curves reach the specified level and yield estimates Z_{add} and Z_{mix} whose variances are not too large. It may sometimes happen that the mixture proportions are chosen without knowledge of the values of A and B. When these are ultimately estimated, the value of f can be calculated from

$$f = \rho_A B / (A + \rho_A B - \rho_A A).$$

4.3   Test of significance

The common test for the difference of two means is based on Student's t distribution. In the usual application of this test there are two sets of sample values: a set of observed values, x_1, x_2 ..., x_m for the random variable X and a set of observations, y_1, y_2, ..., y_n on another random variable Y. (Note, unequal numbers, m and n.) It is assumed that X and Y are normally distributed and have the same variance σ^2, an important aspect of the underlying theory. The true means of X and Y may be different, and the object of the test is to determine whether they are different in a probabilistic sense. For this we use the sample means, $\bar{x}$ and $\bar{y}$ and sample variances $s_x^2 = \sum (x_i - \bar{x})^2 / (m - 1)$, $s_y^2 = \sum (y_i - \bar{y})^2 / (n - 1)$, in a test that computes the value of t, with degrees of freedom $= (m + n - 2)$, from

$$t = \frac{\bar{x} - \bar{y}}{s_p\left(\dfrac{1}{m} + \dfrac{1}{n}\right)^{1/2}} . \qquad (4.5)$$

In this formula s_p is the pooled standard deviation, calculated from the sample standard deviations s_x and s_y as follows:

$$s_p^2 = [(m-1)s_x^2 + (n-1)s_y^2]/[m+n-2]. \qquad (4.6)$$

When the pooled variance, s_p^2, assumed to be the common variance of each random variable, is put under the radical in Equation 4.5, the denominator is $[SE_x^2 + SE_y^2]^{1/2}$.

In our application, the sample means and s_p do not come from enumerated data, as above. Instead, these are derived from curve-fitting procedures. For this reason the quantity t' is calculated from the following equation

$$t' = \frac{\bar{x} - \bar{y}}{[(SE_x)^2 + (SE_y)^2]^{1/2}} . \qquad (4.7)$$

We have denoted this quantity by t' in order to distinguish it from the common form given by Equation 4.5. In the form given by Equation 4.7, there is allowance for the fact that the respective standard errors may be different, but this introduces a complication because t' determined this way is not a t value (from the Student distribution) when m and n are small. In other words, some modification of the test is needed. (Snedecor and Cochran, 6th ed., 1967, pp. 114–116; 8th ed., 1989, pp. 96–97; Daniel, W.W., 5th ed., 1991, p.212; Bliss, C.I., 1967, p. 216.)

In this case we need to compare t' with a quantity that is not directly from the table, but instead is computed from table values t_x and t_y as follows:

$$T = [t_x(SE_x)^2 + t_y(SE_y)^2]/[(SE_x)^2 + (SE_y)^2] \qquad (4.8)$$

where t_x is the tabular value of t based on m-2 degrees of freedom and t_y is the tabular value of t based on n-2 degrees of freedom for the level of significance desired (usually, 95%).

In the application at hand, the values to be compared are the mixture potency, Z_{mix}, and the additive potency, Z_{add} (see Relations 4.3

and 4.4). Because these are lognormally distributed, we actually test $\log (Z_{mix})$ and $\log (Z_{add})$ by applying Equations 4.7 and 4.8.

Toward this end, let $X = \log (Z_{add})$ and $Y = \log (Z_{mix})$, with standard errors, SE_x and SE_y on the log scale. The additive data are derived from $(N_1 + N_2)$ points (sum of points of the constituents) and thus we use d.f. $= N_1 + N_2 - 2$. The mixture curve has n_{mix} points and its d.f. is $n_{mix} - 2$. Using the 95% level we get the t values for these, viz., t_{add} and t_{mix}, from the usual tables for their respective degrees of freedom. We then calculate

$$t' = (X - Y)/[(SE_x)^2 + (SE_y)^2]^{1/2} \qquad (4.9)$$

and

$$T = [t_{add}(SE_x)^2 + t_{mix}(SE_y)^2]/[(SE_x)^2 + (SE_y)^2]. \qquad (4.10)$$

If $|t'| > T$ the difference is significant.

Example: Synergism Between Morphine and Clonidine. Tests of analgesic compounds are frequently conducted in mice whose tails are subjected to a nociceptive stimulus. In one test, hot water provides the stimulus, and the effect is measured as tail withdrawal latency measured in seconds, thereby producing a measure of the antinociceptive effect that is on a continuous scale. Morphine sulfate and clonidine hydrochloride, each antinociceptive in this test, were tested individually and in combination. The data in Table 4.1 show the doses and the effects, measured as percent of the maximum effect. Doses are in μg quantities administered by injection into the subvertebral space, and the combination doses are *sums* of each drug's dose (Tallarida et al., 1997). Table 4.1 contains the results of the statistical analysis that began with linear regression of effect on $\log_{10}$ (dose) for the individual drugs and the combination. The regression equations of effect on log dose are shown along with the D_{50} dose and its logarithm for the individual drugs and the combination.

The combination doses shown in Table 4.1 were derived from the D_{50} values of the individual drugs, denoted (as usual) by A and B in the table. The value $f = 0.5$ was used in calculating the additive total, and, thus, the combination had amounts in proportion to 0.5×5.754 for drug A and 0.5×3.755 for drug B. These are 2.877 and 1.8775, respectively. The sum of these, shown as 4.760, is an additive total amount, Z_{add}, for the effect level selected (50%) and would be expected to give the 50% effect. (Its logarithm, needed later, is 0.678.) In fact, this dose gave the much higher effect 92.04 shown in the table.

Table 4.1. Dose-Effect Data for Morphine SO$_4$ and Clonidine HCl

Clonidine HCl (Drug B)		Morphine SO$_4$ (Drug A)		Combination (Drug C)	
Dose	Effect	Dose	Effect	Dose	Effect
0.800	19.79	1.138	19.67	1.190	38.96
2.667	31.40	3.793	40.32	2.380	65.98
7.998	74.92	11.38	61.91	4.760	92.04
26.66	92.41	37.93	88.52		

Drug A: $Y = 15.64 + 45.21 \log(\text{dose})$, $\log(A) = 0.7600 \pm 0.0234$, $A = 5.754 \pm 0.310$

Drug B: $Y = 20.36 + 51.58 \log(\text{dose})$, $\log(B) = 0.5746 \pm 0.0994$, $B = 3.755 \pm 0.858$

Drug C: $Y = 32.46 + 88.16 \log(\text{dose})$, $\log(Z_{mix}) = 0.1989 \pm 0.00317$, $Z_{mix} = 1.581 \pm 0.01151$

(See linear regression equations in Chapters 1 and 2.)

Reduction of this total dose to half determined the other lower total dose tested, 2.380, and another division by 2 gave 1.190. Each of the total doses preserved the ratio of drug A to drug B such that $p_A = 0.605$ and $p_B = 0.395$. From the values of $SE(\log(A))$ and $SE(\log(B))$ shown, the variances of A and B were calculated using Equation 2.12: $SE(A) = 2.30 \times 5.754 \times 0.0234 = 0.3096$, from which $V(A) = 0.0959$, and $SE(B) = 2.30 \times 3.755 \times 0.0994 = 0.8585$, from which $V(B) = 0.7370$. Since $f = 0.5$, the variance of the additive total is calculated from Equation 4.2: $V(Z_{add}) = (0.5)^2 \times (0.0959) + (0.5)^2 \times (0.7370) = 0.2082$. Thus, we get $SE(Z_{add}) = 0.4563$ and $SE(\log(Z_{add})) = 0.0417$.

With Z_{add}, Z_{mix}, and their standard errors now known, it is possible to test the significance of the difference according to Equations 4.9 and 4.10. The test is actually made on the logarithmic values: 0.678 $\pm$ 0.0417 vs. 0.1989 $\pm$ 0.00317. From Equation 4.9 we get

$$t' = (0.678 - 0.199)/[0.00174 + 0.00001]^{1/2} = 0.479/0.0418 = 11.46.$$

The value of t' is to be compared with T given by Equation 4.10. The table values of t for the additive set uses 6 degrees of freedom and 95%; this is 2.447 (see Table A.6). For the combination (3 points) the degrees of freedom = 1, and thus the table value is 12.706. Hence,

$$T = [(0.0417)^2 \times 2.447 + (0.00317)^2 \times 12.706]/(0.00174 + 0.00001)$$
$$= 2.505.$$

Since $t' > T$ the difference is clearly significant, thereby demonstrating synergism.

It should be noted that nonoverlapping confidence limits for log Z_{add} and log Z_{mix} means that the difference is significant, and this criterion has been used for this purpose. This is a more strict criterion than the assessment based on the modified t-test given here.

4.4   Graphical display with standard errors

It has been previously mentioned that the isobologram is not convenient for statistical analysis. Nevertheless, when a separate statistical analysis has been conducted, as in the preceding section, it may still be desirable to display the results on an isobologram. The statistical analysis leads to the estimated values Z_{add} and Z_{mix} of the respective totals and the standard error of each (square root of variance), as illustrated in the above example. It is therefore possible to display these standard errors as vertical and horizontal segments through the additive point and the mixture point of the isobologram. The half width of each segment indicates the standard error for each constituent and is parallel to the axis representing that constituent as in Figure 4.1. The calculated standard error is that for the total: Z_{add} for the additive and Z_{mix} for the combination. For each total the proportions of the constituents, denoted ρ_A and ρ_B, are known. Thus, standard errors are $\rho_A\ SE(Z_{add})$, $\rho_B SE(Z_{add})$ for the additive point and $\rho_A\ SE(Z_{mix})$, $\rho_B\ SE(Z_{mix})$ for the experimental point. It is interesting to note that for each point the sum of the standard errors in each direction is the standard error of the total. This (unusual) relation follows from the fact that the constituents are in a fixed ratio mixture. (See this chapter's appendix for details.)

It might be supposed that, using Equation 4.1, the standard errors of the constituents in the additive case could be obtained as $f\ SE(A)$ and $(1 - f)\ SE(B)$ because the additive combination contains amounts $f A$ and $(1 - f)B$. That would be incorrect because these are controlled amounts (although based on *estimates* of A and B) that define the combination; as such, fA and $(1 - f)B$ have no error. When these amounts are put together, the total has a variance because the theoretical definition of additivity is based on the true A and B and not the estimates that are used to make the combination.

4.5   The additive total dose: a closer look

Equation 4.1 allows a calculation of the additive total dose in terms of the fractions, f and $1 - f$, and Equation 4.2 calculates its variance. Clearly

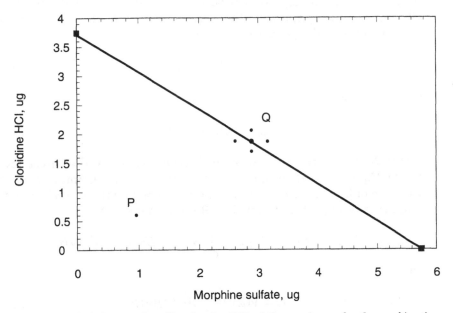

Figure 4.1. Isobologram for effect level = 50% of the maximum for the combinations of morphine sulfate and clonidine HCl in a fixed ratio proportion in which the quantities of the constituents are in proportion to their respective D_{50} values. The solid line is the line of additivity and contains the point Q representing the calculated additivity quantities for this proportional combination. Point P is the combination point determined experimentally with this same proportional mix. The coordinates of point Q are (2.88 ± 0.28, 1.88 ± 0.18) and the coordinates of point P are (0.96 ± 0.007, 0.62 ± 0.004). (Redrawn from Tallarida, R.J., Stone, D.J., and Raffa, R.B. Efficient designs for studying synergistic drug combinations. *Life Sci.* 61:PL417–425, 1997. Used with permission of Elsevier Science.)

these are needed in a test to distinguish additivity from nonadditivity. The literature, however, has not addressed this need with a method for getting these values. As a result, many studies that utilized the isobologram presented the plot with no error estimates. Consequently, the conclusions reached in these studies were based solely on this graphical view. The need for estimates of Z_{add} and its standard error prompted a derivation (Tallarida et al., 1989) that led to formulas for Z_{add}, the total amount (or concentration) in a simply additive combination, and its standard error. In contrast to the simple formulas given in Equations 4.1 and 4.2, derived more recently, the earlier work started by using the proportions, ρ_A and ρ_B, of the combination and the ratio $R = A/B$. This approach led to formulas more complicated than 4.1 and 4.2, especially that for $V(Z_{add})$. We provide the main results of this earlier work here because some aspects will be useful in subsequent discussion in Chapter 5. In that approach the total additive amount was expressed in terms of ρ_A and ρ_B (whose sum = 1) as follows:

$$\rho_A Z_{add}/A + \rho_B Z_{add}/B = 1 \tag{4.11}$$

from which Z_{add} follows as

$$Z_{add} = A/(\rho_A + R \rho_B) \tag{4.12}$$

where $R = A/B$, the ratio of equieffective doses for the effect level. While Equation 4.12 is not very complicated the estimation of the variance of Z_{add} based on this equation is a good deal more complicated (Tallarida et al., 1989; Tallarida, 1992); it is given by

$$V(Z_{add}) = (\rho_A + R \rho_B)^{-2} [V(A) + C E^2 - 2E V(A)/B] \tag{4.13}$$

where

$$C = V(A)/B^2 + A^2 V(B)/B^4 \tag{4.14}$$

and

$$E = \rho_B Z_{add}. \tag{4.15}$$

The above variance calculation, which required the use of the ratio R and an estimation of its variance, is seen to be somewhat more complicated (and probably less accurate) than the expression given in Equation 4.2. The computing form of Z_{add} given by Equation 4.12 is, however, simple enough and gives the same value as that from Equation 4.1. Figure 4.2, showing three lines derived from linear regression and the calculated additive line, displays the main ideas in tests for synergism, additivity, and sub-additivity. The lines represent log dose-effect data from the individual compounds, the additive line, and the mixture line. All doses are totals of the constituents. The additive line is always between the individual compound lines. The position of the mixture line, however, can be either coincident with the additive line or on either side of it. The horizontal line represents the specified effect level, here denoted E*, and its intersection with each of the four lines provides logarithms of A, B, Z_{add} and Z_{mix} as shown. The order relation between Z_{add} and Z_{mix} classifies the nature of the interaction as previously discussed. It should be noted that no aspect of this analysis depends on the lines' being parallel.

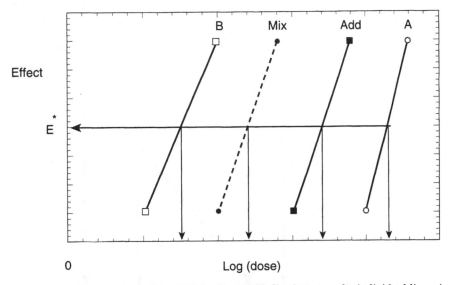

Figure 4.2. The position of the additive line (Add) lies between the individual lines A and B and depends on the proportions of the fixed-ratio combination. The position of the combination line (Mix) determines whether the interaction is super-additive or sub-additive. For the specified level of effect (E^*) the logarithms of B, A, Z_{mix} and Z_{add} are indicated by the vertical arrows. In this case there is synergism ($Z_{mix} < Z_{add}$).

4.6   Changing the effect level

Studies of interactions begin with dose-effect data of each constituent, and, as we have seen, these data are often modeled with regression lines. Also, some effect level (such as 50% of the maximum) that is common to both agents is selected for subsequent analysis. At this level the values of A and B are estimated, along with their variances, and these values are used in determining the proportions of the constituents. In some cases it may be desirable to examine the nature of the interaction at other levels for this same proportioned mixture. If complete dose-effect data are available this is easy enough, provided that there is sufficient precision in the regression lines at the new level. Figure 4.3 illustrates the calculation. Effect vs. dose (on a log scale) shows the original effect level E_1 and a new higher effect level E_2. At the new effect level the equieffective doses (or concentrations) are denoted by A^* and B^* and are calculated from the individual regression equations. The variances of these at the new level, $V(A^*)$ and $V(B^*)$ are also calculable from Equation 2.9. The variance of Z_{add}

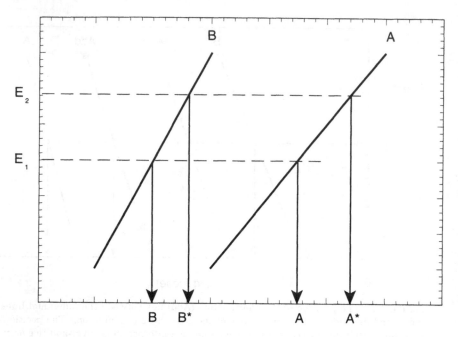

Figure 4.3. Changing the effect level.

at the new level requires the fraction f at this new level as seen in Equation 4.2. While the proportions ρ_A and ρ_B remain the same, changing the effect level changes f since it is now the fraction of A^* that is needed. This new fraction, here denoted by f^*, is calculated from A^*, B^*, and ρ_A from Equation 4.16:

$$f^* = \frac{\rho_A B^*}{A^* + \rho_A B^* - \rho_A A^*}. \qquad (4.16)$$

With f^* now determined from the above, Equations 4.1 and 4.2 can now be used with starred quantities to get Z_{add} and its variance at the new level.

The level that is chosen in this kind of analysis (isobolar, i.e., equieffective comparisons of doses) will usually be near the 50% E_{max} level. It is desirable to have the variances of all dose estimates as small as possible, and the value of the variance of logdose (or dose) in regression analysis depends on how close it is to $\bar{x}$ (see Equation 2.9). Therefore, the dose values used in testing (hence, in analysis) should be those that produce effects near the effect level that is to be used in the analysis. Chapter 5 discusses a method of analysis that is based on the complete mixture and calculated additive regression lines.

4.7   Selecting the drug proportions in a combination study

The choice of the constituent proportions or, equivalently, the selection of f, is somewhat arbitrary. If there is some known reason (mechanistic or other) to guide this selection, then the choice is made. In the absence of this kind of guide it is reasonable to make the choice from an examination of the individual drug data — especially from the variances of the individual D_{50} (or $ED50$) values. In the notation we have employed, f is the fraction of A and $1 - f$ is the fraction of B (A and B are the individual potencies based on the selected effect level — see Equations 4.1 and 4.2). Since the variance of Z_{add} should be as small as possible (to facilitate statistical testing), we can determine the value of f by finding its value that gives a minimum $V(Z_{add})$. This determination is easily accomplished by differentiating $V(Z_{add})$ with respect to f and equating the derivative to zero. This procedure yields

$$f = \frac{V(B)}{V(A) + V(B)}. \qquad (4.17)$$

In many cases the individual variances, $V(A)$ and $V(B)$ are comparable and, if they are equal, the above equation shows that $f = 1/2$. This is a reasonable choice for f even when the variances differ a bit. But when there is a marked difference in the variances that cannot be practically reduced (say, by further testing), and if there is no compelling reason to use some particular proportion, then Equation 4.17 is a rational guide. Figure 4.4 illustrates this for a particular case, that in which the variance of B is twice that of A. It is seen that $f = 2/3$ provides the best choice in this situation.

4.8   Interaction index

When synergism is found $Z_{mix} < Z_{add}$; thus, $Z_{mix} = \alpha\, Z_{add}$ for some value of α that is less than one. The value of α is the interaction index. It is a number that provides a measure of the degree of synergism; i.e., it is an indicator of the dosage reduction that is

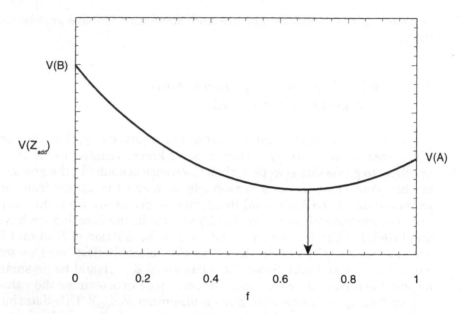

Figure 4.4. The variance of the calculated additive dose depends on the individual variances, $V(A)$ and $V(B)$. In this illustration, $V(B) = 2\ V(A)$, so that the minimum variance of Z_{add} occurs at a proportional combination for which $f = 2/3$.

associated with the particular fixed-ratio combination of the drugs. (It is also an *estimate* since both Z_{mix} and Z_{add} are estimates.) The interaction index is useful in characterizing the synergism and also when it is desired to use the reduced dosages in some situation. For example, in the morphine-clonidine experiment (Table 4.1), we found $Z_{mix} = 1.58$ and $Z_{add} = 4.76$; thus $\alpha = 0.332$ which was obtained with a combination containing 60.5% morphine sulfate. We also saw that the potency ratio of the drugs is $5.754/3.755 = 1.532$ in this test of antinociception. These values can be used to find the reduction in doses as we now illustrate.

Suppose that some experimental situation requires 10 μg of morphine SO_4. We can calculate the needed combination of the constituents that (theoretically) are equivalent to this dose of the opioid. First, we use Equation 4.12 to obtain the additive equivalent of 10 μg of morphine sulfate:

$$\frac{10}{0.605 + (1.532)(0.395)} = 8.263\,.$$

Because of the synergism, we multiply this additive total by the index, $0.332 \times 8.263 = 2.743$ μg. This reduced quantity is the total amount in the synergistic combination of which the morphine component is 1.660 and the clonidine component is 1.083. In these calculations all the values used, and hence the result obtained, are based on the 50% effect level (an isobolar analysis). In Chapter 10 (response surface methods) the analysis is extended to other dose combination ratios and a range of effects, thereby providing a more detailed picture of the synergism.

CHAPTER 4

Appendix

We wish to show that if two random variables, X and Y, are in a fixed proportion, their sum, $Z = X + Y$, has SE given by $SE(Z) = SE(X) + SE(Y)$. To prove this, we square both sides : $SE^2(Z) = SE^2(X) + SE^2(Y) + 2\ SE(X)\ SE(Y)$. But, in general, $SE^2(X + Y) = SE^2(X) + SE^2(Y) + 2\ cov(X, Y)$, for normally distributed variables. Accordingly, we must show that $SE(X)\ SE(Y) = cov\ (X, Y)$. Since X and Y are in a fixed proportion, $Y = \alpha\ X$. Thus, $cov\ (X, Y) = cov\ (X, \alpha X) = \alpha\ cov\ (X, X) = \alpha\ V(X) = \alpha\ SE^2(X)$. Also, $SE(X)\ SE(Y) = SE(X)\ SE(\alpha X) = \alpha\ SE^2(X)$, $= \alpha\ V(X)$, thereby demonstrating the equality.

CHAPTER 4

References

Bliss, C.I. *Statistics in Biology.* McGraw-Hill, New York, 1967.

Daniel, W.W. *Biostatistics: A Foundation for Analysis in the Health Sciences.* Wiley, New York, 1991.

Snedecor, G.W. and Cochran, W.G. *Statistical Methods.* Iowa State University Press, Ames, 1967. 8th ed., 1989.

Tallarida, R.J. Statistical analysis of drug combinations for synergism. *Pain* 49:93–97, 1992.

Tallarida, R.J., Porreca, F., and Cowan, A. Statistical analysis of drug-drug and site-site interactions with isobolograms. *Life Sci.* 45:947–961, 1989.

Tallarida, R.J., Stone, D.J., and Raffa, R.B. Efficient designs for studying synergistic drug combinations. *Life Sci.* 61:PL417–425, 1997.

CHAPTER 5

The Composite Additive Curve

When dose-effect data from two drugs have been obtained, and each is fitted to a linear regression line, the relative potency R at any effect level can be estimated. We now consider how the two data sets and R values can be used to obtain a third curve that represents a simply additive combination for any fixed-ratio combination of the two. The procedure produces a curve that is a composite of the two.

5.1 Construction of the additive curve

The less potent drug is denoted by *drug* 1 and the more potent by *drug 2*. Consider a dose-effect point of drug 1 that has coordinates (log z_1, y) as in Figure 5.1. The effect level y is common to both drugs, and, thus, there is a relative potency R calculable from the curves. R is the ratio of the equivalent doses (drug 1:drug 2) from the curves, as shown in the figure. The combination has proportions, ρ_1 of drug 1 and ρ_2 of drug 2. An additive combination is given by the following (see Equations 4.11, 4.12):

$$Z_{add} = \frac{z_1}{\rho_1 + R\rho_2}. \tag{5.1}$$

Thus, Z_{add} is the sum of both constituents in an *additive combination* with relative potency R, having proportions ρ_1 and ρ_2, and producing the same effect level as the dose of z_1 of drug 1 alone. Since the denominator of Equation 5.1 is greater than 1, Z_{add} is less than z_1. Stated differently, Z_{add} is less than z_1 because the more potent drug (2) is present in the combination. Thus, for all the effect levels produced by drug 1, the combination's additive total is less than the dose of drug 1 acting alone. If the points (log Z_{add}, y) are plotted, the resulting graph is a translation to the left of the original plot because each point is translated by an amount, log $(\rho_1 + R\rho_2)$.

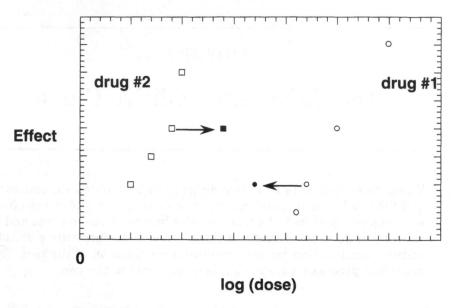

Figure 5.1. Dose-effect data from drug 1 and 2 are plotted. An additive total dose from drug 1 is a lesser quantity, shown as a leftward shift. The more potent drug 2 has an additive total that is a greater quantity, shown here as a rightward shift. The set of shifted points produces an additive composite for the combination in fixed-ratio combination of the constituents.

Now consider drug 2. When it is present in an additive combination with the less potent drug 1, the total in an additive combination is greater than the dose z_2 of drug 2 acting alone that gives the same effect. We have in this case

$$Z_{add} = \frac{z_2}{(\rho_1/R) + \rho_2}. \tag{5.2}$$

When compared to the points of drug 2, log Z_{add} lies to the right of log z_2. (See Figure 5.1). The translated points of both drugs result in a set of points that are the composite of both. It has been shown that the translated points are theoretically not linear, but the departure from linearity is only very slight in most cases studied (Tallarida et al., 1997). Further, the shifted amounts contain a relative potency term (R) that is not known precisely, because it is estimated from the two regression lines. Accordingly a regression line derived from the additive set of points is based on x-values that are not known precisely.

Methods exist to handle bias associated with cases in which the x-values have error (Snedecor and Cochran, 1989; Draper and Smith, 1981), but, as a practical matter (based on numerous tests), there is no serious error when standard regression is applied to the set of translated points (Tallarida et al., 1997) and the error is probably less serious than the common procedure of constraining the lines to parallel.[*] The composite additive set allows the construction of a regression line of additivity for the drug pair and the relative proportions of the constituents of the combination. When an actual combination with this proportional mix is tested we get a second regression line that may be directly compared to the additive regression line.

The following example illustrates the computational details. These data are from the same experiment illustrated in Table 4.1 of Chapter 4. These are experiments with morphine SO_4 and clonidine HCl administered intrathecally to mice that were then tested for antinociception in a test based on tail withdrawal latency (Tallarida et al., 1997). The proportions of the constituents were 0.605 for morphine SO_4 and 0.395 for clonidine HCl. The effect is expressed as the percentage of the maximum effect.

Example. Doses of clonidine (C) and morphine (M) are shown in the first column of Table 5.1 and the effects of these are shown in the last

Table 5.1. Doses and Additive Equivalent

	Dose	Add	Effect
C:	0.800	0.917	19.79
C:	2.667	3.179	31.4
C:	7.998	10.916	74.92
C:	26.66	38.220	92.41
M:	1.138	1.030	19.67
M:	3.793	3.230	40.32
M:	11.38	9.052	61.91
M:	37.93	27.569	88.52

Clonidine: $Y = 51.581 x + 20.055$ $D_{50} = 3.756 \pm 0.859$

Morphine: $Y = 45.215 x + 15.639$ $D_{50} = 5.754 \pm 0.310$

---

[*]The parallel constraint is a common procedure in pharmacologic data analysis, a practice that assumes constant relative potency at all effect levels. This practice has been questioned by Finney (1971) but no practical remedy has been found.

column. An additive combination consisting of 0.605 morphine and 0.395 clonidine would require the total dose ("Add") shown to get the same magnitude of effect. It is seen that the additive totals are greater than the clonidine doses but less than the morphine doses. The additive equivalents are calculated from Equations 5.1 for M and 5.2 for C, using the doses and the values $\rho_1 = 0.605$, $\rho_2 = 0.395$, and the appropriate value of R at each effect level. The R-values were derived from the individual log dose-effect lines whose equations are given at the bottom of the table.

For example, at effect level 31.4, achieved with clonidine dose 2.667, the clonidine line gives $x = 0.2141$ and the morphine line gives $x = 0.3486$. These are log dose values and their difference is log $R = 0.1345$, from which $R = 1.363$ (rounded). Using dose $z_2 = 2.667$ and the values of ρ_1, ρ_2 and R in Equation 5.2, we get

$$Z_{add} = \frac{2.667}{(0.605/1.363) + 0.395} = 3.179$$

as shown in Table 5.1. In other words, a dose of clonidine = 2.667, acting alone, would require 1.363 times this amount of morphine (acting alone) = 3.635 to attain this same effect level. The calculated $Z_{add} = 3.179$ is a total dose of which clonidine is 39.5% = 1.256 and morphine is 60.5% = 1.923. (Note that 1.256/2.667 + 1.923/3.635 = 1) . For the morphine doses and each effect a similar calculation of R is made at the specified effect level and Equation 5.1 is used in computing each of the additive dose equivalents given in Table 5.1.

When all points are translated the set is the additive equivalent. The regression line that is determined from this set is therefore the additive equivalent line for this fixed-ratio combination (Figure 5.2). For each combination ratio that is to be used, there is a different additive line. Accordingly, when an experiment with an actual fixed ratio combination is conducted, its regression line may be compared with that of the calculated additive equivalent line for the same combination. The additive line also provides values of log D_{50}, in this case, 0.676 ± 0.042, which agrees closely with the value 0.678 obtained from Equation 4.1 (see Chapter 4); thus, the log D_{50} values of the actual combination and the calculated additive log D_{50} may be compared. *The construction and use of the additive equivalent line provides an alternate method of getting the additive log D_{50} value,* i.e., in addition to the value determined from Equation 4.1. Tests with numerous drug pairs have shown that the two methods agree very closely as in this

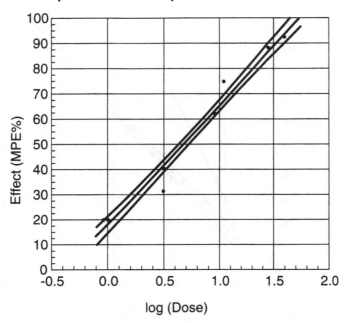

Figure 5.2. The composite regression line (with standard error bands) is calculated from the individual data sets and is given by the equation $Y = 17.35 + 48.33\ x$. From this line, $\log\ (D_{50}) = 0.676 \pm 0.042$. The composite line is based on 60.5% morphine SO_4 and 39.5% clonidine HCl.

example. Figure 5.3 shows the regression line for the three combination doses that were actually tested (data in Table 4.1), along with the additive line calculated for this combination. The composite additive line provides a view of the (total) log dose-effect relation over the entire range of doses used and effects attained with the individual drugs. This composite line allows a comparison with the line derived from an actual combination experiment with this same fixed-ratio proportion and is shown for this example in Figure 5.3.

The importance of the additive line is further illustrated in Figure 5.4 which shows it along with experimental results of a combination experiment (artificial data used). A combination that is synergistic may result in the situation shown in Figure 5.4a. This is synergism over the entire range studied. The graph also illustrates the effect level = 50% of the maximum effect as a horizontal line that intersects to give the log D_{50} doses of the additive and experimental lines. These

Morphine + Clonidine

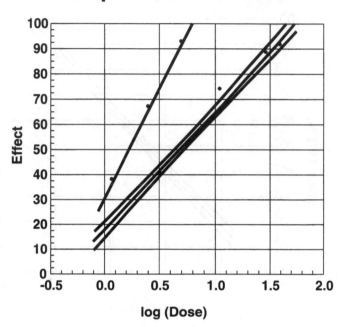

Figure 5.3. Dose effect line (*left*) for the combination of morphine SO_4 (60.5%) and clonidine HCl (39.5%) along with the calculated composite additive line (*right*) shown for the same combination (with standard error bands).

would be statistically compared as described in Chapter 4, Equations 4.6 to 4.10. Another possible outcome is illustrated in Figure 5.4b. In this case the synergism may be significant at the 50% effect level but not at the lesser effect levels. In other words, the synergism is dependent on the total dose in this fixed proportion combination. A third possibility is shown in Figure 5.4c in which the regression lines are nearly coincident. This illustrates *additivity over the entire range* of the tested doses, and Figure 5.4d shows a situation in which the lines intersect at the mid range doses, a case that can hardly be classified as synergistic. In practice each of these situations does occur, so a classification of synergism depends not only on the drugs and the effect measured, but also on the fixed ratio combination and the total dose in the combination.

These illustrations point out the desirability of having additional methods for determining and classifying combinations that depart from additivity. The application of the *t*-test at the effect level chosen

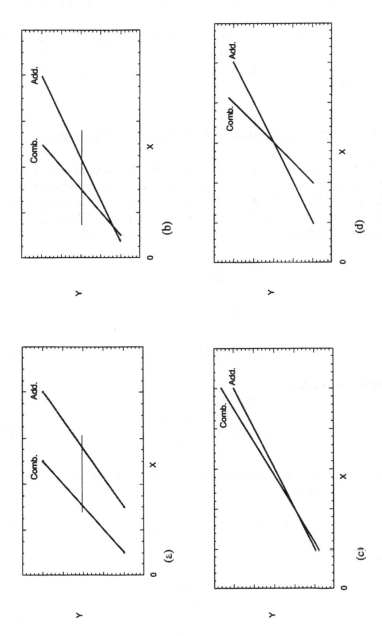

Figure 5.4. Some possible examples of the combination regression line and the additive regression line for the same proportions of constituents. The plots in (a) and (b) show a difference in the combination and additive total doses over an appreciable dose range, and this difference at an effect level in the midrange of the plots (horizontal lines) may be significant. Case (c) shows that there is no departure from additivity, whereas (d) is a more complicated finding showing additivity in the midrange and a divergence that would not be clearly classified at other combination doses.

(e.g., 50% of the maximum) provides only one indication and is clear only in situations such as those shown in Figure 5.4a and b. In actual work, the additive regression line and the line obtained from experiment should be compared to assess whether synergism, if it is found at some mid range effect, extends to other dose levels. The F-distribution provides a convenient statistic for distinguishing whether the two lines differ significantly.

5.2   Test for distinguishing two regression lines

Our application is to the line of additivity and the actual combination line. The method, however, is general for any two regression lines. First, the points from both data sets are used, *without distinguishing between each*, to determine the mean values $\bar{x}$ and $\bar{y}$. We then calculate terms, denoted SS_t and SS_p, from the formulas below.

$$S_{xx} = \sum (x_i - \bar{x})^2 \qquad\qquad (5.3)$$

$$S_{xy} = \sum (x_i - \bar{x})(y_i - \bar{y}) \qquad\qquad (5.4)$$

$$S_{yy} = \sum (y_i - \bar{y})^2 \qquad\qquad (5.5)$$

From these we get SS_t:

$$SS_t = S_{yy} - \frac{(S_{xy})^2}{S_{xx}}. \qquad\qquad (5.6)$$

To get SS_p we use the residual sum of squares from *each* line, $SS_{res(1)}$ and $SS_{res(2)}$, and add them

$$SS_p = SS_{res(1)} + SS_{res(2\cdot)} \qquad\qquad (5.7)$$

From these we calculate F:

$$F = \frac{\dfrac{SS_t - SS_p}{2}}{\dfrac{SS_p}{N_1 + N_2 - 4}} \qquad\qquad (5.8)$$

Degrees of freedom for F are 2 (across) and $(N_1 + N_2 - 4)$ (down). In our application, line 1 is the composite additive line, which is derived from the sum of the points of both drugs; that sum gives N_1. The value of N_2 equals the number of data points in the actual combination experiment.

Example. Comparing Additive and Experimental Regression Lines. Table 5.2 shows the results of a combination experiment with two similarly acting compounds. In this experiment each compound was first given alone in five doses and produced mean effects (% of maximum) as shown in the table. Results of linear regression analysis show that for drug #1, $D_{50} = 100.0$ and for drug #2, $D_{50} = 65.13$. The combination dose proportions were taken to be the same as the D_{50} values; thus, 100.0:65.13. Therefore a typical combination dose, based on $f = 1/2$, contained $1/2(100) + 1/2 (65.13) = 82.56$ (a total that is expected to give a 50% effect in an additive combination). All other combination doses retained this ratio and had total amounts, 10.32, 20.64, ... 165.13. (See "Combination Data" in Table 5.2.) The proportion of drug #1 is 0.6056 and that of drug #2 is 0.3944. For this choice the additive $D_{50} = 82.56$ and is displayed in the table as $Z_{add(2)}$.

The table also includes as composite parameters the shifted dose and log dose values corresponding to each effect of the individual drugs, thereby resulting in 10 points that comprise the additive composite data set. Regression on this set gave $Z_{add} = 81.04$, shown in the Table as $Z_{add(c)}$, a value that agrees well with $Z_{add(2)}$ calculated above. The agreement is more striking for the logarithmic values, 1.91 and 1.92 on which the analysis is based. The experiment with the actual combination having these proportions produced a $D_{50} = 17.94$, a number significantly less than the additive. This finding suggests super-additivity, and the difference (based on log values) was significant, as noted by the calculated t' and tabular T values. The composite line and the experimental line were compared using Equation 5.8 which requires values for SS_t, SS_p, N_1 and N_2. The merged data gave the value $SS_t = 8872.1$, while the summed residuals gave $SS_p = 637.8$. The value $N_1 = 10$ for the composite line and $N_2 = 5$ for the experimental line; substitution in Equation 5.8 gives $F = 71.00$. This exceeds the table value 3.98 (degrees of freedom 2, 11 of Table A.9 at 0.05 level). This result means that the additive and combination lines are significantly different, a conclusion that seems evident from the equations of these two lines.

Table 5.2.   Combination Analysis: Comparing the Additive and
Experimental Regression Lines

Compound 1

Dose	Log (dose)	Effect (%)
50	1.699	2.5
75	1.875	18
100	2.000	35
125	2.097	70
150	2.176	95

Eqn: $Y = 192.0\ x - 334.1$
Log D_{50} = 2.00 ± 0.031
D_{50} = 100.0 ± 7.19

Compound 2

Dose	Log (dose)	Effect (%)
20	1.301	6
40	1.602	24
80	1.903	52
120	2.079	78
160	2.204	92

Eqn: $Y = 96.69\ x - 125.4$
Log D_{50} = 1.814 ± 0.030
D_{50} = 65.13 ± 4.55

Composite Data

f = 0.500
P_1 = 0.6056
$Z_{add(C)}$ = 81.04 ± 3.85
$Z_{add(2)}$ = 82.56 ± 4.25

Dose	Log(dose)	Effect (%)
29.992	1.477	2.5
31.821	1.503	6
50.355	1.702	18
58.468	1.767	24
75.268	1.877	35
100.252	2.001	52
115.343	2.062	70
127.204	2.105	78
153.514	2.186	92
156.009	2.193	95

Table 5.2.   (Continued)Combination Analysis: Comparing the Additive and Experimental Regression Lines

$$Eqn: \quad Y = 127.99\,x + -194.30$$
$$\bar{x} = 1.887$$
$$\bar{y} = 47.25$$

SS_{tot} = 11019
SS_{res} = 555.9 $\log D_{50}$ = 1.909 ± 0.021
SS_{reg} = 10463 D_{50} = 81.04 ± 3.85

Combination Data

f = 0.500
P_1 = 0.6056

Dose	Log(dose)	Effect (%)
10.320	1.014	32
20.640	1.315	55
41.280	1.616	75
82.560	1.917	92
165.130	2.218	100

$$Eqn: \quad Y = 57.47\,x + -22.05$$
$$\bar{x} = 1.616$$
$$\bar{y} = 70.80$$

SS_{tot} = 3074.8
SS_{res} = 81.91 $\log D_{50}$ = 1.254 ± 0.053
SS_{reg} = 2993 D_{50} = 17.94 ± 2.20

Results

F = 71.00
t' = 11.44
T = 3.067

CHAPTER 5

References

Draper, N. and Smith, H. *Applied Regression Analysis*, 2nd ed., John Wiley, 1981.

Finney, D.J. *Probit Analysis*, 3rd ed. Cambridge, 1971.

Snedecor, G.W. and Cochran, W.G., *Statistical Methods.* Iowa State University Press, Ames, 1967. 8th ed., 1989.

Tallarida, R.J., Stone, D.J., and Raffa, R.B. Efficient designs for studying synergistic drug combinations. *Life Sci.* 61:PL417–425, 1997.

CHAPTER 6

Quantal Dose-Response Data: Probit and Logit Analysis

We have seen that the effects of drugs and chemicals are often expressed on a continuous scale. Muscle tension, blood pressure, and measures of time duration that are used in analgesic tests are examples. In other situations a drug dose is given and we look for some sign or endpoint. For example, did the animal stretch after receiving an irritating intraperitoneal injection? Did the animal show a response to some hot or cold stimulus? Did the animal die after receiving the drug? In these cases, either the subject shows the response or does not show the response. These are examples of binary outcomes, and we can record the proportion of the sample that displays the sign and, thus, the proportion that did not. The proportion data are coupled to the dose of drug that is intended to inhibit the response (or show the response). Thus, these are all-or-none, or *quantal*, data. The data set consists of (dose, proportion responding).

Proportion data do not have a uniform variance, i.e., as the proportion (p) changes (with changing dose) the variance changes. For large numbers (n) this variance is given by $p(1 - p)/n$. The probit method of linear regression adjusts for this non-constant variance through the application of weights, as we will describe in this chapter. Another procedure useful for proportion data is the log odds transformation, i.e., we convert each p_i to the quantity, $\ln [p_i/(1 - p_i)]$ called the "logit." This, too, has a variance that is not constant; thus weights are used. This method, known as "logit analysis" is discussed at the end of this chapter.

6.1 Probit analysis

We now consider test situations in which we divide the population tested with a specific drug dose into responders and non-responders based on a particular endpoint or characteristic. This is a quantal situation. Thus, if n subjects or animals are tested at a specific dose, then either 0, 1, 2, ..., n, experience the effect. This number of responders r divided by n gives the proportion p that respond; thus, $p = r/n$ and multiplying p by 100 gives the percentage that respond. The association of the proportion of responders with the dose produces quantal dose-effect data. The proportion (or percentage) is usually plotted against the dose or the logarithm of the dose, and an appropriate smooth curve is drawn to fit the data. The sigmoidal curve of Figure 6.1 is an example of a smooth curve that is typical of this plot. It is desirable to have the data produce a straight line, for then linear regression can be used to get the best fitting straight line. Toward this end several transformations have been tried. One that is especially suitable is embodied in a calculation algorithm called *probit analysis*. In this procedure, the proportion responding to each dose is transformed into a number called a "probit." The graph of probit against log(dose) produces points that often display a linear trend, and, therefore, this graph is modeled as a straight line using "weighted" linear regression. Before presenting the details of this linear regression procedure, we discuss the probit and its relation to the normal distribution.

The cumulative probability function P for a normal distribution with mean 0 and variance 1 is well known. It represents the probability

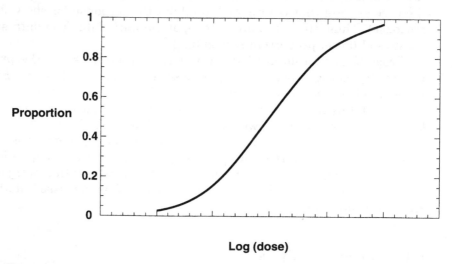

Figure 6.1. S-shaped curve representing the proportion plotted against log dose. This shape is typical of those obtained in quantal experiments and has been modeled in relation to the standard normal curve and also according to the logistic curve.

that some random variable has a value that is less than or equal to some number. This number, denoted here by Y, is termed the normal equivalent deviate. P is given by the integral

$$P = \frac{1}{\sqrt{(2\pi)}} \int_{-\infty}^{Y} \exp(-u^2/2) du \tag{6.1}$$

and represents the probability that the random variable is less than or equal to Y. The integrand in the above integral is a bell-shaped curve. Graphically, P is the area under this curve from negative infinity to Y. The area under the total curve, from minus infinity to plus infinity, is unity. If P is plotted against Y, the curve is sigmoidal, as shown in Figure 6.2. This shape is similar to that obtained from quantal dose-effect curves in which the proportion of respondents is plotted against the log(dose). To the extent that the quantal dose-effect curve has the shape of the cumulative probability function, it follows that the relation between the log(dose) and the normal equivalent deviate is linear, a concept recognized by Gaddum (1933). Bliss (1934) replaced the normal equivalent deviate by a quantity that increased it by 5 and called it a probit. Thus, the probit Y is given by

$$P = \frac{1}{\sqrt{(2\pi)}} \int_{-\infty}^{Y-5} \exp(-u^2/2) du . \tag{6.2}$$

From Equation 6.2 it is seen that $Y = 5$ corresponds to $P = 0.5$. A table of probits for specified values of P is given in the appendix (Table A.8), and a graph of the probit-percentage relation is given in Figure 6.3. Plotting the probit against the log(dose) is straightforward, but the regression technique requires weights in order to stabilize the unequal variances that accompany proportions and, hence, probits. Accordingly all the summations used in the simple linear regression formulas are modified to include weights (w_i) that must be computed in this regression procedure. (Weighted regression is discussed in Chapter 3.)

The first step in probit analysis is the conversion of each proportion (or percentage) to a probit, using Table A.8. It is worth noting *there are no probits for 0 and 100%*. Thus, these values of response, if they occur, are not used initially. The proportion (p_i) of responder among the n_i tested at each log dose value (x_i) is calculated as the number of responders divided by the number n_i of subjects tested at this dose.

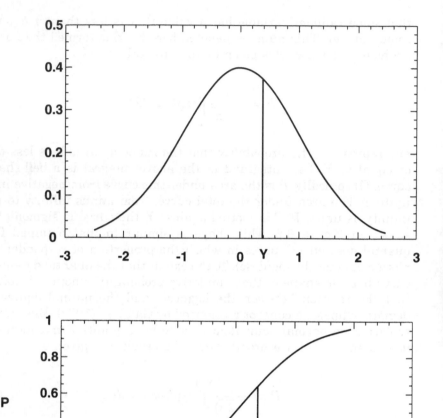

Figure 6.2. Upper graph is the standard normal distribution curve; the area under the total curve is one. The area under the curve and lying to the left of the vertical line at abscissa = Y represents some proportion P. The lower graph shows P, plotted as the ordinate against Y, which results in the S-shaped (sigmoidal) curve.

Each proportion is converted to a probit value. Some notation is needed. We shall denote the probit of proportion p_i by the symbol y_i' and the log dose value that produced this by x_i. The set of points (x_i, y_i') are then first used in a simple regression procedure (see Equations 2.3 and 2.4) to produce the initial regression line. Note that the index

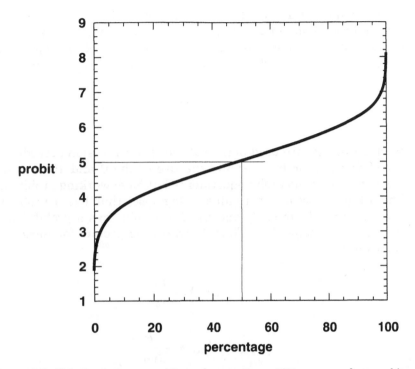

Figure 6.3. Relation between probits and percentages; 50% corresponds to probit = 5.

i refers to the ith dose, n_i are tested at that dose, and there are N distinct doses; thus, $i = 1, 2, ..., N$. The value of the probit *on the line* (the expected probit) is here denoted by Y_i and the proportion corresponding to it will be denoted P_i. These are used in the calculation of weighting factors w_i from the following:

$$w_i = \frac{n_i f_i^2}{P_i(1 - P_i)} \tag{6.3}$$

where

$$f_i = \frac{1}{\sqrt{2\pi}} \exp\left[-\frac{1}{2}(Y_i - 5)^2\right]. \tag{6.4}$$

It should be noted that the calculation of weights uses values from the line.

The values of w_i, which involve f_i, are used in the construction of a second regression line, but this second line no longer uses the probits of the original proportions. Instead the original set of proportions, p_i, are used to obtain *working probits*, y_i, that are calculated from

$$y_i = Y_i + \frac{p_i - P_i}{f_i}. \tag{6.5}$$

Working probits are used in the subsequent regression procedure. The use of working probits permits the use of the 0 and 100% response points that have no probit equivalents but have working probit values. The 0% point occurs at a value of log(dose) that has a probit value from the line, denoted Y_0, and the 100% point has a probit from this initial line, denoted Y_{100}. Thus, the working probits for these special values are

$$y_0 = Y_0 - \frac{P_0}{f_0} \tag{6.6}$$

$$y_{100} = Y_{100} + \frac{1 - P_{100}}{f_{100}}. \tag{6.7}$$

Because weights are obtained from values on the line, it is seen that these "special" points have weights, as do all the others. The complete set of working probits and their weights are used to calculate a second regression line

$$Y = a + bx. \tag{6.8}$$

The values of a and b are determined from the following formulas that incorporate weights with summation over the N values of i:

$$b = \frac{\sum w_i(x_i - \bar{x})(y_i - \bar{y})}{\sum w_i(x_i - \bar{x})^2} \tag{6.9}$$

and

$$a = \bar{y} - b\bar{x} \tag{6.10}$$

where

$$\bar{x} = \sum w_i x_i / \sum w_i \qquad (6.11)$$

$$\bar{y} = \sum w_i y_i / \sum w_i . \qquad (6.12)$$

This second (improved) regression line is now used to get another set of weights and another set of working probits for the original x_i, p_i values, and these are paired with the x_i values to get a third regression line, $Y = a + bx$, computed from the above formulas. The process continues as an iterative procedure. Two or three cycles of calculation usually produce a satisfactory fit. (Theoretically, the maximum likelihood estimate is the limit to which these estimated lines tend in an infinite process.)

Prior to the widespread availability of computers the labor involved in these calculations impeded the use of the probit method. Several approximate methods were developed that used various graphical procedures and nomograms. One approximate graphical method was developed by Litchfield and Wilcoxon (1949) and became routinely used. The appendix to this chapter contains additional discussion of this graphical method.

The probit regression line obtained from the iterative method described here serves the same function as the curve of empirical proportion responding vs. log(dose), except that the proportions 0 and 1 have no corresponding empirical probits. The working probit values that are derived from the line for these values permit their incorporation into the analysis. The probit regression line has the advantage of being linear and can therefore be analyzed from formulas for weighted linear regression. The equation is simple, e.g., the log (*ED50*) is the x value from the line at which $Y = 5$. Similarly, the x-value for any other proportional response can be obtained by substituting its corresponding probit for Y in the straight line equation and solving for x. But it is necessary to obtain error estimates of log (*ED50*), the other parameters, and the other measures of potency. These are readily calculated in probit analysis as we now show.

6.2   Precision in probit calculations

The estimated intercept (a) and slope (b) of the probit regression line have variances (square of standard error) given by

$$V(a) = \frac{1}{\sum w_i} + \frac{\bar{x}^2}{\sum w_i(x_i - \bar{x})^2} \tag{6.13}$$

and

$$V(b) = \frac{1}{\sum w_i(x_i - \bar{x})^2}. \tag{6.14}$$

At any value of x the probit estimate from the regression equation has a variance

$$V(Y) = \frac{1}{\sum w_i} + \frac{(x - \bar{x})^2}{\sum w_i(x - \bar{x})^2}. \tag{6.15}$$

The mean value, $\bar{y}$, has a variance given by

$$V(\bar{y}) = \frac{1}{\sum w_i}. \tag{6.16}$$

Confidence limits are calculated using values from the normal distribution; e.g., 1.96 (for 95% confidence limits) multiplies the standard error (square root of variance) to give a quantity that is added and subtracted from the estimated parameter values. There is special interest in the confidence limits for log ($ED50$) which is estimated from the final regression line as the x-value for $Y = 5$, and, thus it is $x^* = (5 - a)/b$. Because x^* is the ratio of estimated quantities, a precise variance is not available. An approximate value is given by

$$V(x^*) = \frac{1}{b^2}\left[\frac{1}{\sum w_i} + \frac{(x^* - \bar{x})^2}{\sum w_i(x_i - \bar{x})^2}\right]. \tag{6.17}$$

The above variance formula is actually applicable to any x^* value, e.g., log ($ED20$), or log ($ED80$). A confidence interval based on this variance is approximate. A true confidence interval for x^*, e.g., the confidence interval of log ($ED50$), is computed from

$$x^* + \frac{g}{(1-g)}(x^* - \bar{x}) \pm \frac{st}{b(1-g)}\left\{\frac{1-g}{\sum w_i} + \frac{(x^* - \bar{x})^2}{\sum w_i(x_i - \bar{x})^2}\right\}^{1/2} \tag{6.18}$$

where

$$g = \frac{s^2 t^2}{b^2 \sum w_i (x_i - \bar{x})^2}.$$ (6.19)

It is seen that these confidence limits are unequally spaced to the left and right of x^*. The theory on which the probit method is based requires that $s = 1$ and that t has a value from the normal distribution, such as 1.96 for the 95% confidence interval. However, heterogeneity of the data, indicated by too large a value of the residual sum of squares, requires additional considerations that we now explain.

In this and other regression procedures, there are uncontrolled and unknown factors that disperse the points about the line in a random way. A measure of the dispersion is afforded by the residual sum of squares, $\sum w_i (y_i - Y_i)^2$. This is a random variable that has the χ^2 distribution with degrees of freedom $= N - 2$. If testing reveals a value of SS_{res} that exceeds the tabular entry (Table A.7) then it becomes necessary to incorporate the factor $s^2 = SS_{res}/(N - 2)$ into all variance estimates; i.e., all the above variances are multiplied by s^2. In this case, it is also necessary to replace the value from the normal distribution (e.g., 1.96) with the appropriate value of t from Student's distribution (Table A.6) in the calculation of confidence limits. The number of degrees of freedom for t is $N - 2$.

> **Example.** The quantal data (Table 6.1) were obtained in a study of acetaminophen (Raffa et al., 1999) in which mice received intrathecal doses (μg) and were studied in the mouse abdominal constriction test. The table shows the final weights and working probits as well as the original (empirical probits) corresponding to the proportions that responded to each dose used.

6.3   The composite additive probit line

In the previous chapter we discussed the additive composite regression line; that line was obtained by translating log dose values. We now discuss how the composite probit line of additivity is calculated from quantal data. The calculation begins with the final probit lines of the individual compounds. These allow a determination of the relative potency R for every empirical proportion p_i. Even though working probits define the lines, the composite additive line is *initially* made up of empirical proportions as we now describe.

Table 6.1. Probit Analysis of Dose-Response Data

Dose	Log(dose)	Weight	# Test	# Resp	Prop	Probit	W-probit
45.350	1.657	18.09	50	5	0.100	3.718	3.720
90.700	1.958	11.79	20	7	0.350	4.615	4.616
151.170	2.179	11.41	18	11	0.611	5.282	5.280
226.760	2.356	5.684	10	6	0.600	5.253	5.231

$Y = 2.548x - 0.4457$

$\bar{x} = 1.944$

$\bar{y} = 4.507$

$r = 0.975$

$Sxx = 3.091$

$Sxy = 7.878$

$s = 1$

slope $= 2.548 \pm 0.083$

y-int $= -0.4457 \pm 1.115$

$SStot = 21.13$

$SSres = 1.056$

$SSreg = 20.07$

$\log ED50 = 2.137 \pm 0.072$

$ED50 = 137.2 \pm 22.6$

Data: Raffa et al., 1999.

Consider a point from drug 1 (the right-most set). For dose z its coordinates are (log z_i, p_i). To determine the magnitude of the leftward shift, we use relative potency R at the vertical probit level that corresponds to proportion p_i. This p_i is converted to a probit in order to find R from the two lines. The leftward shift is a translation from log z_i to [log z_i − log $(\rho_1 + R\rho_2)$]; the proportion is the same. (Note the difference between lower case p_i and the Greek symbols ρ_1 and ρ_2 that denote the proportions of the combination.) In this expression ρ_1 is the fraction of the combination that is drug 1, and $\rho_2 = 1 - \rho_1$ is the fraction that is drug 2. If there is a 0% point or a 100% point, there is no corresponding probit. In such cases the final working probits are used to get R and, hence, the shift. But once the shift is made, the empirical proportion, 0% or 100%, is paired with the shifted log dose value. The result of shifting is to produce the set of (log dose, proportion) points. This same procedure is applied to the data of drug 2 except that the points are shifted to the right by an amount $\log(\rho_1/R + \rho_2)$. This final set of left and right translated points have coordinates (log dose, proportion) and may contain 0 and 100% proportions.

A completely new probit analysis is made on the translated data points. This produces a new set of weights in the usual iterative procedure through several cycles. The final line, along with the final working probits and final weights, must be retained because these are needed in comparing the final composite additive probit line with the mixture's final probit line.

Example. Acetaminophen, a well-known analgesic, was studied in combination with an experimental compound that displayed analgesic activity in the mouse abdominal constriction test. Data for the individual compounds consist of the proportion responding (binary outcome) among the number tested and were therefore subjected to a probit regression analysis. The data and the resulting probit equation of each compound are given in Table 6.2. From these equations it was possible to determine the relative potency R at each level of probit (Y) corresponding to the observed proportion (p) responding at each dose. It was desired to obtain the additive composite probit line for a combination containing 87.49% acetaminophen based on mass; thus $\rho_1 = 0.8749$ and $\rho_2 = 0.1251$. At each effect level, the additive equivalent log dose was a translation (on the log scale) of the acetaminophen log(dose) to the left by amount log $(\rho_1 + R\rho_2)$ and of the experimental compound to the right by amount $\log(\rho_1/R + \rho_2)$. These translated quantities allowed a determination of the additive equivalent dose (Z_{add}). The resulting nine additive equivalent doses and their proportions (p) produced the composite probit line given in Table 6.2. From this composite line the additive $ED50$ (and its logarithm) were determined.

Table 6.2. Dose-Effect Data for Acetaminophen and an Experimental Compound: Construction of the Composite Additive Line*

Drug 1. Acetaminophen (Probit equation $Y = 2.566\ x - 0.298$)

Dose	$x = \log(\text{dose})$	n	p	y'	R	$\log(\rho_1 + R\rho_2)$	Z_{add}
30	1.477	10	0.1	3.72	7.820	0.2679	16.184
60	1.778	10	0.2	4.16	7.523	0.2591	33.029
100	2.0	10	0.4	4.75	7.143	0.2476	56.546
200	2.301	10	0.7	5.52	6.675	0.2330	116.95
300	2.477	10	0.9	6.28	6.244	0.2191	181.092

Drug 2. Experimental Compound (Probit Equation: $Y = 2.337\ x + 2.148$)

Dose	$x = \log(\text{dose})$	n	p	y'	R	$\log(\rho_1/R + \rho_2)$	Z_{add}
3.0	0.4771	10	0.1	3.72	7.820	-0.6253	12.659
10	1.00	10	0.2	4.16	7.523	-0.6173	41.428
20	1.301	10	0.4	4.75	7.143	-0.6063	80.779
30	1.477	7	1.0	6.42#	6.167	-0.5735	112.331

Composite Line. (Probit Equation: $Y = 2.423\ x + 0.5837$);
$\text{Log}(ED50) = 1.822 \pm 0.0641; ED50 = 66.41 \pm 9.79$

* p: proportion responding; n: number tested; y': probit of p; R: relative potency; Z_{add}: additive equivalent dose; $\rho_1 = 0.8749$: fraction of total that is drug 1; $\rho_2 = 1 - \rho_1 = 0.1251$.

The value 6.42 is the working probit and was used in calculating R (hence, the shift) while the observed proportion, $p = 1$, was used in the calculation of the composite probit line. Z_{add} is obtained from x and the shifted amount in column 7. The composite line's equation is based on values of p and $\log(Z_{add})$ in a separate probit analysis (retaining more decimal places than shown above). The values of $\log(ED50)$ (and $ED50$) are derived from this equation and, thus, are the calculated additive values. Doses are mg/kg, p.o.

Data courtesy of R.B. Raffa and A. Cowan.

6.4 Testing for synergism

When the additive *ED50* has been calculated from the composite line (or is calculated from Equations 4.1 and 4.2 and probit analysis on the two compounds) this *ED50* is tested against the combination *ED50* with the *t*-test given in Equations 4.9 and 4.10. (The test is on the logarithms of the *ED50*s.) This comparison, based on the 50% level, distinguishes between synergism and additivity. But the composite line, as we previously saw, allows a comparison over the entire range of effects.

6.5 Comparing the composite additive line and the actual combination line

The composite additive regression line is derived from the two individual probit regression lines by shifting the data points as previously described. That line is now compared with the line obtained from actual combination data in the same fixed ratio combination used in calculating the additive composite line. (In Chapter 5 a similar comparison is made on two ordinary regression lines.) In our example the combination contained 87.49% acetaminophen ($\rho_1 = 0.8749$). The comparison involves the use of the final working probits and weights of each. Table 6.3 shows these values for the additive composite line. Table 6.4 shows these values for the combination data and also gives the raw data for the combination in this fixed

Table 6.3. Working Probits and Weights for Additive Composite Regression

	x	y	w
Composite			
	1.103	3.937	1.952
	1.209	3.751	2.734
	1.519	4.163	5.215
	1.617	4.192	5.818
	1.752	4.747	6.299
	1.908	4.741	6.268
	2.051	6.401	3.982
	2.068	5.523	5.590
	2.258	6.255	4.199

Table 6.4. Combination Dose-Effect Data and Probit
Results (for $\rho_l = 0.8749$)

Data	
Total dose	No. respond/No. tested
17.49	0/10
26.24	3/10
34.99	5/10
52.48	9/10
69.98	10/10

Probit analysis results		
log dose	w-probit	weight
x	y	w
1.243	2.542	1.218
1.419	4.498	5.103
1.544	4.999	6.329
1.720	6.272	3.037
1.845	7.674	0.763

Combination Probit Equation: $Y = 7.205\, x - 5.997$; log $(ED50)$
$= 1.526 \pm 0.0342$; $ED50 = 33.605 \pm 2.645$

proportion ($\rho_1 = 0.8749$). These combination data have been slightly
modified to enhance this illustration.

The F-test is used to determine whether the mixture probit line is
different from the composite additive line. The final working probits
of each, and their final weights, are used in this comparison. The test
uses calculated quantities SS_t and SS_p.

To get SS_t: Without distinguishing the two lines, we take every
point from both and determine the mean values

$$\bar{x} = \frac{\sum w_i x_i}{\sum w_i} \tag{6.20}$$

and

$$\bar{y} = \frac{\sum w_i y_i}{\sum w_i} \tag{6.21}$$

where x is log(dose) values and y is the final working probit. Then
calculate

$$A_t = \sum w_i(x_i - \bar{x})^2 \qquad (6.22)$$

$$B_t = \sum w_i(x_i - \bar{x})(y_i - \bar{y}) \qquad (6.23)$$

$$C_t = \sum w_i(y_i - \bar{y})^2 \qquad (6.24)$$

and

$$SS_t = C_t - \frac{(B_t)^2}{A_t}. \qquad (6.25)$$

To get SS_p: Add the residual sum of squares of both the additive and mixture lines

$$SS_p = {}_{(add)}SS_{res} + {}_{(mix)}SS_{res}. \qquad (6.26)$$

The quantities SS_t and SS_p are used to calculate F:

$$F = [(SS_t - SS_p)/2] / [SS_p/(N_{add} + N_{mix} - 4)]. \qquad (6.27)$$

Degrees of freedom are 2 (across) and $N_{add} + N_{mix} - 4$ (down). A significant difference requires that the calculated F exceed the tabular at the significance level chosen (e.g., 95%). Table 6.3 shows the working probits (y), log dose (x) and weights (w) for the composite additive regression and Table 6.4 gives these for the combination regression for acetaminophen and the experimental analgesic. The probit equation for the combination is also given, along with *ED50* and its logarithm. A comparison of the additive composite and combination regressions needs the residual sum of squares for each. These are $_{add}SS_{res} = 6.136$ and $_{comb}SS_{res} = 0.846$. Thus, $SS_p = 6.982$. Additionally, we calculate the other terms needed in the comparison using Equations 6.22–6.27:

$A_t = 5.229;$ $B_t = 12.155;$ $C_t = 49.49$, from which F is calculated:

$$F = [(21.235 - 6.982)/2] / (6.982/10) = 10.21.$$

The tabular value (d.f. 2, 10) at the 0.05 significance level is 4.10. Thus the regression lines are significantly different. The log *ED50* values of the additive composite and combination lines were also used in the

t-test described by Equations 4.7 and 4.8, and gave $t' = 4.07$ and $T = 2.54$, thereby confirming the significance shown by the F-test.

6.6   A closer look at probits

The log(dose) values, denoted x_i, have a mean value μ and a standard deviation σ. The standard normal curve (used in probit analysis) has an abscissa $u = (x - \mu)/\sigma$. The probit corresponding the proportion is $u + 5$; thus, probit $= 5 + (x - \mu)/\sigma$. It follows that the plot of probit against log(dose) is a straight line with slope $= 1/\sigma$. This connection between the slope and the standard deviation has an application in methods for comparing two compounds with probit lines. The log doses of both compounds are assumed to be normally distributed and, frequently, with the same (or nearly the same) standard deviation. Accordingly, the probit lines of effect vs. log(dose) are expected to be parallel. Many therapeutic (and toxic) effects of two compounds are compared with parallel lines.

6.7   Testing two probit regression lines for parallelism

Probit analysis uses weights; thus some of the terms involved in regression formulas need to have new definitions that incorporate the weights. For example, S_{xx}, previously introduced in Chapter 2, now denotes $\Sigma w_i(x_i - \bar{x})^2$. Similarly, in probit analysis we define $S_{xy} = \Sigma w_i(x_i - \bar{x})(y_i - \bar{y})$ and $S_{yy} = \Sigma w_i(y_i - \bar{y})^2$, where the summation is over the N points of the line. For two lines there are N_1 points for line 1 and N_2 points of line 2. Our goal here is to examine two probit regression lines for parallelism. The two lines will have been determined from their final working probits (the y values above). The test of parallelism uses the F-statistic and certain calculations that we now describe.

The residual sum of squares, SS_{res}, is determined for each line and these are summed to form the quantity denoted P:

$$P = {}_1SS_{res} + {}_2SS_{res}. \tag{6.28}$$

We further need the quantities calculated from each data set:

$$A = {}_1S_{xx} + {}_2S_{xx}, \quad B = {}_1S_{xy} + {}_2S_{xy}, \quad C = {}_1S_{yy} + {}_2S_{yy}$$

and

$$M = C - B^2/A.$$

The value of F is computed from

$$F = [M - P] / [P/(N_1 + N_2 - 4)]. \qquad (6.29)$$

This calculated F is compared with the tabular value for $d.f. = 1$ (across) and $N_1 + N_2 - 4$ (down). If the calculated F is less than the tabular value, the lines do not differ significantly from parallel, and a common slope b_c is calculated from the formula

$$b_c = \frac{{}_1S_{xy} + {}_2S_{xy}}{{}_1S_{xx} + {}_2S_{xx}}. \qquad (6.30)$$

The individual probit regression lines are given by

$$Y_1 = \bar{y}_1 + b_c(x - \bar{x}_1) \qquad (6.31)$$

and

$$Y_2 = \bar{y}_2 + b_c(x - \bar{x}_2). \qquad (6.32)$$

(See example, Table 6.5.) Because these lines are constrained to be parallel, the residual sum of squares (SS_{res}) should be calculated for each. If either shows heterogeneity, we calculate the pooled error variance

$$s_p^2 = ({}_1SS_{res} + {}_2SS_{res})/(N_1 + N_2 - 3). \qquad (6.33)$$

The quantity s_p^2 is used to get the following variances that are needed subsequently:

$$V(\bar{y}_1) = s_p^2/{}_1\Sigma w_i, \; V(\bar{y}_2) = s_p^2/{}_2\Sigma w_i, \; V(b_c) = s_p^2/({}_1S_{xx} + {}_2S_{xx}) \quad (6.34)$$

If testing shows that there is no heterogeneity, then all s_p^2 terms are replaced by unity.

Table 6.5. Parallel Line Analysis

Data Set: Drug 1

Dose	Log(dose)	Weight	# Test	# Resp	Prop	Probit	W-probit
100.0	2.000	4.442	10	2	0.200	4.158	4.168
200.0	2.301	5.703	10	3	0.300	4.476	4.476
400.0	2.602	9.505	15	6	0.400	4.747	4.748
800.0	2.903	12.26	20	11	0.550	5.126	5.121
1000.0	3.000	8.829	15	12	0.800	5.842	5.803

$Y = 1.446x + 1.124$
$\bar{X}mean = 2.671$
$\bar{Y}mean = 4.987$

$r = 0.91$
$Sxx = 4.442$
$Sxy = 6.425$
$s = 1$

slope $= 1.446 \pm 0.0743$
y-int $= 1.124 \pm 1.277$

$SStot = 11.10$
$SSres = 1.809$
$SSreg = 9.293$

$\log ED50 = 2.680 \pm 0.108$
$ED50 = 478.4 \pm 119.2$

Data Set: Drug 2

Dose	Log(dose)	Weight	# Test	# Resp	Prop	Probit	W-probit
2.0	0.301	2.708	10	1	0.100	3.718	3.754
4.0	0.602	4.686	10	2	0.200	4.158	4.160

8.0	0.903	9.193	15	5	0.333	4.569	4.571
16.0	1.204	12.42	20	11	0.550	5.126	5.124
32.0	1.505	7.315	15	13	0.867	6.111	6.081

$Y = 1.946x + 2.919$

$\bar{x} = 1.044$

$\bar{y} = 4.950$

$r = 0.974$

$S_{xx} = 4.466$

$S_{xy} = 8.692$

$s = 1$

$\text{slope} = 1.946 \pm 0.0785$

$\text{y-int} = 2.919 \pm 0.521$

$SStot = 17.84$

$SSres = 0.9290$

$SSreg = 16.91$

$P = 2.738$

$A = 8.908$

$B = 15.12$

$C = 28.95$

$\log ED50 = 1.069 \pm 0.0855$

$ED50 = 11.72 \pm 2.305$

$M = 28.947 - (15.117)^2/8.908$

$= 3.293$

$F = (3.293 - 2.738)/(2.738/6)$

$= 1.216$

$b_c = (6.425 + 8.692)/(4.442 + 4.466)$

$= 1.697$

$Y = 4.987 + 1.697(x - 2.671)$ } equations of

$Y = 4.950 + 1.697(x - 1.044)$ } parallel lines.

Probits are based on original proportions; weights and working probits (W-probit) are from the final regression lines. Test of parallelism uses calculated F and the tabular value (= 5.99, for 95% and d.f. = 1, 6), indicating in this case that the slopes are not significantly different and allowing calculation of the common slope b_c.

6.8   Constant relative potency in probit analysis

Parallel regression lines indicate that the relative potency of the two compounds is a constant; i.e., at all levels of effect the relative potency is the same. Accordingly, the difference between the equally effective x values (log dose) is the same. This distance, denoted here by W, is given by

$$W = (\bar{x}_1 - \bar{x}_2) - (\bar{y}_1 - \bar{y}_2)/b_c \qquad (6.35)$$

so that the relative potency is given by

$$R = 10^W. \qquad (6.36)$$

Confidence limits for W are given by the following (Finney, 1971):

$$W + \frac{g}{(1-g)}(W - \bar{x}_1 + \bar{x}_2) \pm$$
$$\frac{t}{b_c(1-g)}\langle(1-g)\{V(\bar{y}_1) + V(\bar{y}_2)\} + (W - \bar{x}_1 + \bar{x}_2)^2 V(b_c)\rangle^{1/2}. \qquad (6.37)$$

In this formula, $g = t^2 V(b_c)/b_c^2$ and t is the normal deviate (=1.96 for 95%), but if a heterogeneity factor (s_p^2) is incorporated into the variance terms, as previously described, then t has a value from Student's distribution with degrees of freedom $N_1 + N_2 - 3$. The lower and upper confidence limits, W_l and W_u, yield the lower and upper confidence limits of R:

$$R_l = 10^{W_l} \quad \text{and} \quad R_u = 10^{W_u}. \qquad (6.38)$$

Note that if g is neglected, these confidence limits are

$$W \pm \frac{t}{b_c}[V(\bar{y}_1) + V(\bar{y}_2) + (W - \bar{x}_1 + \bar{x}_2)^2 V(b_c)]^{1/2}. \qquad (6.39)$$

The term multiplying t in the equation above is seen to be the square root of the "variance" of W (standard error).

6.9   Parallel line analysis of combined drug action

Comparisons of the potency of two compounds and probit analysis of the combined action of the two have traditionally been made under the assumption of a constant relative potency. When the individual dose-effect relations are based on this assumption their linear log(dose)-effect curves are parallel. The common slope (previously denoted b_c) is here denoted b.

Under the assumption of parallelism, the dose-effect relation of drug 1 is

$$Y_1 = a_1 + b \log (z) \tag{6.40}$$

and that for drug 2 is

$$Y_2 = a_2 + b \log (z) \tag{6.41}$$

Parallelism, indicated by the common slope b, means a constant relative potency, R; hence, equieffective doses, z_1 of drug 1 and z_2 of drug 2, are related as $z_1/z_2 = R$. If doses z_1 and z_2 are present together, the total dose can be expressed as an equivalent of drug 1, viz, $z_1 + R z_2$, and the effect of this combination is then given by the equation for drug 1:

$$Y = a_1 + b \log (z_1 + R z_2). \tag{6.42}$$

This expression of equivalence defines additivity, i.e., the drugs contribute to the effect in a way that is consistent with their relative potency. If the individual doses are in a fixed proportion, ρ_1 and ρ_2 of the *total dose* (z), then Equation 6.42 becomes

$$Y = a_1 + b \log (z) + b \log (\rho_1 + R \rho_2) \tag{6.43}$$

Figure 6.4 shows the dose-effect graph of drug 1 and the additive graph for the combination plotted on the same axes. It is seen that the additive curve is elevated in relation to the curve of drug 1. Alternatively it can be described as a translation (shift) to the left.

The curve of additivity can also be derived by expressing the combination dose with the use of drug 2 as the reference drug. In this case the equation of drug 2 is used and the total dose is written, $z_2 + z_1/R$. Thus the equation is given by

$$Y = a_2 + b \log (z_2 + z_1/R). \tag{6.44}$$

and, in terms of the *total dose* z, the relation is

$$Y = a_2 + b \log (z) + b \log (\rho_1/R + \rho_2). \tag{6.45}$$

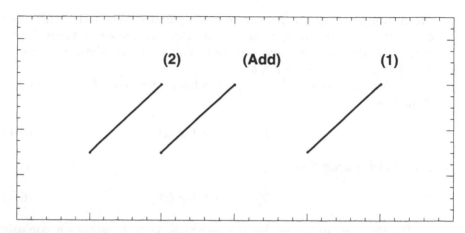

Figure 6.4. In analyses in which the constituent curves display parallelism, the line of additivity is parallel to these and lies between the regression lines of drugs 1 and 2. The precise location of the additive line depends on the relative proportions of drugs 1 and 2. See Equation 6.43.

The last term in Equation 6.45 is negative, so this form of the additive curve has less elevation than the curve of drug 2 alone (Figure 6.4). Alternatively, this curve can be viewed as a translation to the right of drug 2's dose-effect curve. (It should be noted that Equations 6.43 and 6.45 are equivalent; either form describes the line of additivity.)

The results of the analysis in this section illustrate how one can view the regression line of additivity in relation to the individual drug lines. We showed earlier that the additive total dose–effect relation does not really depend on parallelism, i.e., one could produce this relation from lines that are not parallel simply by using the value of R at each level of effect. Nevertheless, the parallel line analysis is often useful.

6.10   Testing for additivity: parallel constraint and probit analysis

The previous section considered the individual drugs under the assumption of a constant relative potency and showed how one can calculate the additive regression line of a fixed ratio combination of the two. That line, given by Equation 6.43, is expressed in terms of the total dose in the combination. When actual combination data are available, this third set of values (total dose, effect) is used in the calculation of the common slope. The goal is to compare the calculated additive line with the actual combination line.

The data from the individual drugs and from the fixed ratio combination (proportions ρ_1 and $\rho_2 = (1 - \rho_1)$ of the total) provide the information needed to detect a departure from additivity. Under the assumption of parallelism, these have the same slope b calculated from the data for drug 1, 2, and the combination (3), the latter described by

$$Y_3 = a_3 + b \log (z). \qquad (6.46)$$

The common slope is calculated from the three data sets

$$b = \frac{{}_1S_{xy} + {}_2S_{xy} + {}_3S_{xy}}{{}_1S_{xx} + {}_2S_{xx} + {}_3S_{xx}} \qquad (6.47)$$

and the intercept (a) of each line is computed from this common slope and its own mean values $\bar{x}$ and $\bar{y}$ as $a = \bar{y} - b\bar{x}$.

Equations 6.40 and 6.41 apply to the individual drugs. With slope b now determined, the relative potency R can be computed from

$$\log (R) = (a_2 - a_1)/b \qquad (6.48)$$

while Equation 6.43 (or 6.45) gives the additive equation in terms of the total dose. We shall use the form given by Equation 6.43 for the additive line. The horizontal distance between the additive line and the combination line given by Equation 6.46 is a measure of the departure from additivity. This distance is calculated from quantities that have error and this fact has to be considered in making this calculation. From Equations 6.43 and 6.46 this distance is given by the following:

$$|D| = (a_3 - a_1)/b - \log(\rho_1 + R\rho_2). \qquad (6.49)$$

Its variance is neatly expressed in a formula given by Finney (1971):

$$V(D) = \left[\frac{\lambda^2}{\sum\limits_1 w} + \frac{(1-\lambda)^2}{\sum\limits_2 w} + \frac{1}{\sum\limits_3 w} + \frac{\{\lambda\bar{y}_1 + (1-\lambda)\bar{y}_2 - \bar{y}_3\}^2}{b^2 \sum S_{xx}} \right] / b^2 \qquad (6.50)$$

where

$$\lambda = \frac{\rho_1}{\rho_1 + R\rho_2}.$$ (6.51)

In this expression, the summation (ΣS_{xx}) in the denominator of the fourth term in the bracket is over the three, whereas the w terms are summed from the three individual data sets. In this entire analysis it is assumed that the three data sets have been tested for parallelism. A confidence interval based on this variance is $D \pm 1.96 \, [V(D)]^{1/2}$. An interval that does does not include 0 indicates a departure from additivity.

6.11   Logit analysis

We have seen that many quantal dose-response curves have a sigmoid shape when the proportion is plotted against log dose and that the transformation of proportions to probits will often be an acceptable linear model of these data. The probit is based on the area under the standard normal curve. Other linearizing transformations can be used to model the same data. One that is in widespread use is based on the logistic function, which is also sigmoidal and given by

$$P = \frac{1}{1 + e^{-(a+bx)}}$$ (6.52)

where P is the proportion and x is the log dose. If the proportion P is transformed to a quantity $L = \ln [P/(1 - P)]$ it is seen that Equation 6.52 becomes

$$L = a + bx.$$ (6.53)

L is called the *logit* corresponding to P. Figure 6.5 shows the linear plot that results when a logistic curve is plotted with logits. To the extent that actual log dose-response data are well fitted to the logistic curve, the logit plot of the same data will be well fitted to a line obtained by regression of logit on log dose.

As in other regression procedures, the values of a and b are estimates of parameters that are found by a procedure that minimizes the sum of the squared deviations of the empirical logit values ℓ_i from

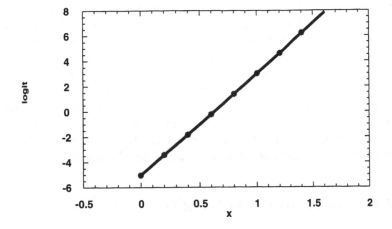

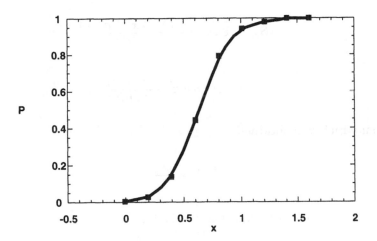

Figure 6.5. Upper graph is a plot of *logit* against x (log dose) corresponding to the plot of proportion against log dose shown in the lower graph.

the expected logits given by Equation 6.53. The regression procedure uses weights whose values depend on the empirical proportions, p_i, and the number of objects, n_i, in the group on which the proportion is obtained. As in probit analysis, or in any other weighted linear regression, the weights are used to stabilize the variances. Unlike probit analysis, however, the algorithm for finding the weights is simpler in logit analysis. Further, the procedure that calculates the values of a and b in logit analysis is not iterative. These two facts make the entire procedure simpler to carry out than is the case in probit analysis. Both methods give very nearly the same results for log *ED50* and its standard error. Why, then, should we not always use this method? Because of a limitation of the logit procedure, namely, that there are no logits corresponding to proportions 0 or 1. Thus, when much of the data are in groups that have these extreme responses, the method of logits should not be used.

6.12   Calculations with logits

The empirical proportions, denoted p_i, are converted to logits, $\ell_i = \log_e(p_i/(1-p_i))$, and weighting factors w_i are calculated as $w_i = p_i(1-p_i)$ to obtain S_{xy} and S_{xx} from the following:

$$S_{xy} = \Sigma nwx\ell - \frac{(\Sigma nwx)(\Sigma nw\ell)}{\Sigma nw} \tag{6.54}$$

$$S_{xx} = \Sigma nwx^2 - \frac{(\Sigma nwx)^2}{(\Sigma nw)} \tag{6.55}$$

from which b is obtained

$$b = \frac{S_{xy}}{S_{xx}}. \tag{6.56}$$

The mean values of x and ℓ are calculated as

$$\bar{x} = \frac{\Sigma nwx}{\Sigma nw} \qquad \bar{\ell} = \frac{\Sigma nw\ell}{\Sigma nw} \tag{6.57}$$

from which we get the parameter estimate

$$a = \bar{\ell} - b\bar{x}. \tag{6.58}$$

The log *ED50*, denoted x', corresponds to $L = 0$; thus it is given by $x' = -a/b$, or

$$x' = \log ED50 = \bar{x} - \frac{\bar{\ell}}{b}. \tag{6.59}$$

Variances of log *ED50* and b are given by

$$V(x') = \frac{1}{b^2}\left[\frac{1}{\Sigma nw} + \frac{(x' - \bar{x})^2}{S_{xx}}\right] \tag{6.60}$$

and

$$V(b) = \frac{1}{S_{xx}} \tag{6.61}$$

from which the standard errors are obtained:

$$SE(x') = [V(x')]^{1/2} \tag{6.62}$$

$$SE(b) = [V(b)]^{1/2}. \tag{6.63}$$

Table 6.6 shows sample calculation with data on acetaminophen.

Table 6.6. Example. Dose (z) and Proportional Response (r/n) for Intrathecal Acetaminophen in Mice: Logit Analysis

x	r	n	l	w	z (µg)	r/n	nw	nwx	nwx^2	$nwxl$	nwl
1.656	5	50	-2.197	0.09	45.35	5/50	4.50	7.45	12.34	-16.37	-9.89
1.958	7	20	-0.619	0.2275	90.70	7/20	4.55	8.91	17.44	-5.52	-2.82
2.179	11	18	0.452	0.2376	151.17	11/18	4.28	9.32	20.31	4.21	1.93
2.355	6	10	0.4055	0.24	226.76	6/10	2.40	5.65	13.31	2.29	0.97
							15.73	31.33	63.40	-15.39	-9.81

$\bar{l} = -0.623$ $\bar{x} = 1.99$ $b = 4.22$ $\log ED50 = 2.14 \pm 0.069$

$S_{xy} = 4.135$ $S_{xx} = 0.979$ $a = -9.03$

Raffa et al., 1999; see also Table 6.1.

CHAPTER 6

Appendix

Method of Litchfield and Wilcoxon

Because the probit method is lengthy and iterative, it was not used widely before the availability of computers. Accordingly, Litchfield and Wilcoxon (1949) developed an approximate graphical procedure that used nomograms to facilitate the calculation. The main idea of the method is the construction of the first probit regression line (probit vs. log dose) by converting proportions, other than 0 or 1, to probits. This is a standard (unweighted) line that is used to correct for the 0 and 100% points. The needed weights enter in a subtle way. These are calculated at 3 proportions: 0.16, 0.50 and 0.84. The number of animals tested that gave responses between 16 and 84% are denoted by N, and this number is divided by 3 and assigned to 16%, 50%, and 84% for the calculation of weights (see Equations 6.3 and 6.4). With this choice of n_i and proportions, $(\sum w_i)^{1/2} = 0.7106\ N^{1/2}$. A function S, whose common logarithm $\approx 1/$slope, gives an approximate standard error of log $ED50$ (see Equation 6.17) as log $S/0.7106\ N^{1/2}$. Confidence limits (95%) are $\pm 1.96 \times$ the standard error, which here is $\pm((1.96)/(0.7106\sqrt{N}))$ log $S \approx \pm((2.76$ log $S)/\sqrt{N})$. The antilog $= S^{2.76/\sqrt{N}}$ is the multiplier of the $ED50$ to give the upper confidence limit and is a divisor of $ED50$ to get the lower confidence limit. A detailed discussion, without the nomogram, is given by Tallarida and Murray (1987).

CHAPTER 6

References

Bliss, C.I. The method of probits. *Science* 79:38–39, 1934, and a correction, *Science* 79:409–410, 1934.

Finney, D.J. *Probit Analysis,* 3rd ed. Cambridge University Press, Cambridge, 1971.

Gaddum, J.H. Reports on biological standards, III. Methods of biological assay depending on the quantal response. *Spec. Rep. Ser. Med. Res. Coun. London,* no. 183, 1933.

Litchfield, J.T. and Wilcoxon, F. A simplified method of evaluating dose-effect experiments. *J. Pharmacol. Exp. Ther.* 95:99–113, 1949.

Raffa, R.B., Stone, D.J. and Tallarida, R.J. (abstract, reporting preliminary results) Antinociceptive self-synergy between spinal and supraspinal acetaminophen (paracetamol). 9th World Congress on Pain, Vienna, 1999.

Tallarida, R.J. and Murray, R.B. *Manual of Pharmacologic Calculations with Computer Programs,* 2nd ed. Springer-Verlag, New York, 1987.

CHAPTER 7

Analysis of Drug Combinations Over a Range of Drug Ratios

The combination of two agonist drugs will produce either additive or nonadditive action in a given test. In most testing situations, the focus is on the effect at some particular level, such as 50% of the maximum effect, and a determination of the combination dose that gives this effect level. Various fixed-ratio combinations are used, and some or all of these combinations often show simple additivity. Synergism is much less common. When a departure from additivity is found, however, there is interest in determining whether this finding also applies to other fixed ratio combinations. In one of the earliest demonstrations of the isobologram, that involving chloral hydrate and alcohol (see Chapter 1), it was shown that some combinations were additive, while others were super-additive (synergistic). The isobologram was helpful in visualizing the combinations that gave these results but could not, in itself, confirm this graphical view.

Figure 7.1 demonstrates the typical situation to which we are referring. In this idealized isobologram two sets of points (X and Y) are labeled and these form the basis of our discussion. It is assumed that all data are combinations of drugs A and B that are found, by testing, to give the same level of effect (such as 50% of the maximum). Intercept values are, of course, the quantities of the individual drugs (each acting alone) that give the effect—in this case, 20 dose units for drug A and 12 dose units for the more potent drug B.

The isobologram suggests that combinations **X** are super-additive, while combinations **Y** are additive or, possibly, sub-additive. Each point (combination) will have been statistically tested for additivity, and it is assumed in this example that at least some of the points in set **X** show departures from additivity; the display of points suggests continuity. In other words, there would seem to be no abrupt transition from super-additive to sub-additive. Yet, it is quite likely that the points that are only slightly off the "line" of additivity would not

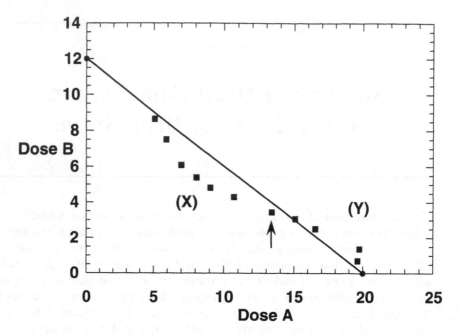

Figure 7.1. Combination doses; the arrow points to a dose pair that is referred to Figure 7.2.

individually differ significantly from additive. In the absence of a mechanism to explain why the two different fixed-ratio combinations show these apparently different interactions, or precisely where the demarcation from additivity to nonadditivity occurs, we can approach the question with modeling equations that allow parameter estimation: we will use a procedure that fits each of the data sets to an appropriate equation that applies over some continuous set of dose ratios. This concept is described using the notation and equations discussed in Chapter 4.

7.1   Fraction plot

From Equation 4.1, $Z_{add} = f A + (1 - f)B$, where the additive total dose, Z_{add}, is expressed in terms of the fraction f of the D_{50} of drug 1, denoted A, and the fraction $(1 - f)$ of the D_{50} of drug 2, denoted B. (Of course, the effect level can be something other than the 50% level, in which case A and B are the doses for that particular effect.) Each fixed-ratio combination gives the value of f. When the proportion ρ

of drug 1 defines the combination ratio, the values of f and ρ are related: $f = \rho B/(A + \rho B - \rho A)$. The combination's effective total dose for this f value (corresponding to proportion ρ) is denoted Z_{mix} and $Z_{mix} = \alpha\, Z_{add}$, where α is the interaction index. If the index value is less than 1, there is synergism, and if it is greater than 1, there is sub-additivity. If $\alpha = 1$, then the interaction is additive.

In our example (Figure 7.1), with $A = 20$ and $B = 12$, the additive relation is given by $Z_{add} = 20\,f + 12\,(1 - f)$. This relation, plotted in Figure 7.2, is a straight line. This kind of plot, in which the total dose Z_t is plotted against fraction f, provides another way of viewing the additivity condition and corresponds to the line of additivity of the isobologram. In contrast to the isobologram, this plot has the controlled variable f on the abscissa and the total combination dose on the ordinate. Actual combination *total doses* are represented as ordinate values for each fixed ratio combination that is now defined by the value of fraction f which spans the interval 0 to 1. Points significantly below the line denote super-additivity whereas points above denote sub-additivity.

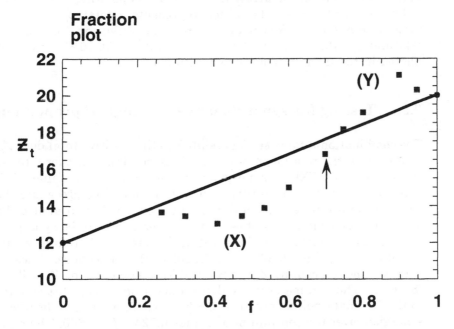

Figure 7.2. Fraction plot corresponding to the isobologram of Figure 7.1; the line indicates additivity. The arrow is for the fraction of drug A corresponding to the combination identified in Figure 7.1. (See text for calculation details.) Z_t represents the total dose in the combination.

The line of additivity of the isobologram of Figure 7.1 is transformed into the line of Figure 7.2, and the individual dose pairs that gave the 50% effect provide the data points, now plotted as total dose, Z_t, against fraction f. The plot of Figure 7.2, referred to here as a *fraction plot*, conveys the same visual information as the isobologram and has the added advantage of allowing statistical analysis. For example, the standard error of the additive line (computed from Equation 4.2 as the square root) at any value of f is easily placed above and below the line and appears as in Figure 7.3.

The construction of the fraction plot is straightforward. For any actual dose pair that is tested in a fixed ratio mixture, the proportion that is drug A and the proportion that is drug B are known in advance. If individual doses, not in a fixed proportion, have been used and it is determined that some combination (a, b) gives the specified effect, then the combination proportion $\rho = a/(a + b)$. This proportion is used, along with the individual $D_{50's}$ (or $ED50's$) A and B, in the formula: $f = \rho B/(A + \rho B - \rho A)$. The sum of a and b gives the total Z_t, and the plot is easily made. For example, the arrow in Figure 7.1 is pointing to the combination $a = 13.36$, $b = 3.44$, which represents a total $Z_t = 16.8$ and proportion $\rho = 0.795$. We calculate f from the above equation, using $A = 20$ and $B = 12$, and get $f = 0.699$. The point (0.699, 16.8) is therefore plotted in the fraction plot (shown with arrow).

7.2   Testing for synergism over a range of proportions

The combination total dose Z_t is related to the additive total dose Z_{add} according to the relation $Z_t = \alpha Z_{add}$. It is possible, therefore, to test the set of points (X) for synergism by determining the value of the index α. This test requires fitting the set of points in a procedure that produces an estimate of α. In this illustration it will be assumed that all but the two end points of set X have been shown to be synergistic using the test procedures discussed in Chapter 4. Therefore, we use the other five points ($0.324 \leq f \leq 0.600$) in this procedure. Since the additive line is given by $Z_{add} = 8 f + 12$, the equation for Z_t is $Z_t = \alpha (8 f + 12)$. The parameter value determined from fitting this equation to the five data points gave $\alpha = 0.876 \pm 0.013$, a value indicative of synergism over the continuum of values $0.324 \leq f \leq 0.600$. The corresponding range of proportions (of drug A) are 0.444 to 0.714. The value of α in this example is not indicative of pronounced synergism, but the value is significantly less than unity on this interval. It is interesting to note that when all the proportions of this combination were

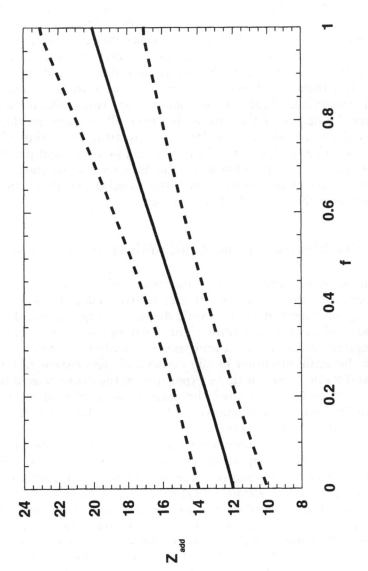

Figure 7.3. Fraction plot of Figure 7.2, showing the additive line, $Z_{add} \pm S.E.$, calculated from Equation 4.2 with $V(A) = 9$ and $V(B) = 4$.

tested (not including the intercept points), the value of α was found to be 0.964 ± 0.025, a value not significantly different from unity.

Although only a discrete set of combinations were tested, the five points that are synergistic produce a curve fit over the continuum of values that are defined by the extreme points of this five-point set. This is so in regression models in which some smooth curve is used to represent the data points. This fact has a special relevance in actual tests for distinguishing nonadditivity from additivity in drug combination experiments. In these experiments, it is possible to test only discrete proportions of the combination, yet one would like to be able to assess the nature of the interaction over all proportions that lie between those actually tested. Hence, estimating the value of the interaction index in this kind of curve-fitting is useful and practical. This determination is possible when the data are transformed to the fraction plot and is not possible with the isobologram. It is this fact that motivated the use of the fraction plot.

7.3   Combinations of acetaminophen and tramadol

Acetaminophen and tramadol are analgesics with efficacies evident in both human and animal studies. It was desired to determine whether combinations of the two agents would display synergism and, if so, in what range of fixed-ratio combinations. Tests in mice were conducted that employed acetaminophen and tramadol hydrochloride that were assessed for antinociception in the abdominal constriction test (Tallarida and Raffa, 1996). In these experiments, the drugs were administered orally and, 30 min later, the animals were injected (i.p.) with acetylcholine bromide, a substance that results in abdominal constriction in the nondrugged animal.

The drug or drug combination efficacy was determined by the absence of writhing during an observation period following injection. From these tests, that employed a number of fixed-ratio combinations, the values of individual $ED50$s and the combination $ED50$ were determined. The latter is based on the sum of the constituent quantities, thereby providing the values of Z_t for each proportion ρ that was employed. The individual $ED50$s were 164.93 ± 24.5 mg/kg, p.o., for acetaminophen (drug A) and 5.52 ± 0.40 mg/kg, p.o. for tramadol HCl. Thus, $A = 164.93$ and $B = 5.52$, and these, along with the proportions allowed a calculation of f for each proportion. Table 7.1 contains the pertinent values and includes the calculated additive $ED50$, denoted $Z_{add,}$ for each combination. Each value of Z_t was derived from a probit

Table 7.1. Values of f and ρ representing various fixed-ratio combinations of acetaminophen and tramadol HCl in the mouse abdominal constriction test. ρ is the proportion that is acetaminophen, and $Z_t = ED50$, the total quantity (mg/kg, p.o.) of the drugs that gave a protective response in 50% of the animals. The calculated additive $ED50$, denoted Z_{add}, is also shown.

f	Z_t	ρ	Z_{add}
3.7500e-05	6.96	0.001	5.53
0.000345	6.90	0.0099	5.58
0.00165	6.78	0.047	5.79
0.0110	10.4	0.25	7.28
0.0324	7.54	0.5	10.7
0.0912	18.9	0.75	20.1
0.143	29.4	0.833	27.9
0.160	27.5	0.851	31.0
0.389	49.9	0.95	67.5
0.621	62.9	0.98	105
0.768	112	0.99	128
0.869	130	0.995	144
0.930	96.0	0.9975	156
0.963	77.7	0.9987	160
0.982	125	0.9994	160

regression analysis of the dose-effect data for the particular proportion and is, therefore, a mean value obtained from that analysis. The standard errors have been omitted in the table in the interest of clarity.

The entries in Table 7.1 have been divided into two groups. In all the entries in the bottom group $Z_t < Z_{add}$. Not all of these were significantly different due to some scatter in the data that produced larger standard errors. In the top group there is no clear trend; in fact, most entries show either additivity or possible sub-additivity. These data suggest the existence of a trend in which additivity becomes super-additivity for the larger proportions (larger proportions of acetaminophen in the combination). Accordingly, the data in the lower half of the table were analyzed in a linear regression of Z_t on f to determine the interaction index α. The equation of the additive line is $Z_{add} = 159.4\,f + 5.52$. Thus the data for Z_t were fitted to $Z_t = \alpha\,Z_{add}$ and gave $\alpha = 0.708 \pm 0.056$, a value indicative of synergism for the set of proportions, 0.851 to 0.999.

CHAPTER 7

Reference

Tallarida, R.J. and Raffa, R.B. Testing for synergism over a range of fixed-ratio drug combinations: replacing the isobologram. *Life Sci.* 58:PL23–28, 1996.

Analysis of a Single
Dose Combination

When a single dose combination of two agonists is administered it is possible to calculate the expected additive effect. This calculation requires that the individual drug dose-response curves be known. This expected effect may then be compared to the effect that is observed experimentally. An assessment of this kind, based on a single combination, is usually not sufficient to classify the drug interaction as additive or nonadditive. For that we need to employ several doses of a fixed-ratio combination and use the more extensive procedures discussed in the previous chapters. The single dose analysis presented here, however, does provide an estimate of the additive effect of a single combination, but it should be regarded as merely a guide to a more complete study. The isobologram is not useful in this determination because that plot is applicable only to a designated effect and that is precisely what we are seeking here.

8.1   Constant relative potency

We denote the two drugs by A and B, the latter being the more potent. The doses of each when acting alone are denoted A and B, respectively. The simplest case is that in which the relative potency $R = A/B$ is the same at all levels of effect. In this case a dose combination consisting of dose a of drug A and b of drug B is easily expressed as an equivalent of either drug.

$$a + R\,b = A_{eq} \qquad (8.1)$$

or

$$b + a/R = B_{eq}. \qquad (8.2)$$

This condition of constant R is exemplified in individual dose-effect relations given by $E = E_{max}A/(A + C_A)$ and $E = E_{max}B/(B + C_B)$. These are hyperbolic dose-effect curves that have the same maximum, E_{max}. The constancy of R in this case is readily obtained by equating effects, and this leads to $R = C_A/C_B$. In this case, and in other cases in which R is constant, the equivalent dose of either drug for combination (a, b) is obtained from Equation 8.1 or 8.2. This equivalent dose is inserted into the dose-effect relation of the reference drug. For example, if A is the reference drug, then Equation 8.1 applies and the effect of the combination is

$$E_{comb} = E_{max}A_{eq}/(A_{eq} + C_A) \tag{8.3}$$

Example. Let the dose-effect relations of two drugs be given by the following:

$$E = 100 \ A/(A + 50) \text{ and } E = 100 \ B/(B + 20)$$

These are hyperbolic curves that have a common maximum = 100 units. We wish to determine the expected (additive) effect of a combination consisting of $a = 40$, $b = 10$.

We first calculate $C_A/C_B = 50/20 = 5/2$. Thus, the given combination is equivalent to $40 + (5/2) (10) = 65$ of drug A alone. This value is used to get the effect level from $E = (100)(65)/(65 + 50) = 56.52$. It is easily calculated that the dose of B alone that gives this effect is $B = 26$. The additivity of the combination (40,10) is confirmed from the sum, 40/65 + 10/26, which is unity.

8.2   Variable relative potency

When the relative potency of the two agonists changes with the effect level, the calculation of the additive equivalent of a combination (a, b) is more complicated. This would occur, for example, where both drugs were described by hyperbolic dose-effect relations having different maxima. Variable potency would also apply if two linear log dose-effect relations have different slopes. (Of course, if the slopes were the same the relative potency would be constant.) Each of these cases is illustrated here.

Hyperbolas with different maxima

We denote the maximum effect of drug A by E_A and that of drug B by E_B. The individual equations are given by $E = E_A A/(A + C_A)$ and $E = E_B B/(B + C_B)$. Let us take drug B as the higher efficacy drug, i.e., $E_B > E_A$. Over the *range of effects that are common to both drugs* we may equate the effects given by the above equations and solve simultaneously with the additive relation $a/A + b/B = 1$. We shall accomplish this by eliminating A and solving for B. From the additivity condition, Equation 1.3, $A = a\,B/(B - b)$, and the equality of effects we get

$$\frac{E_A\left(\dfrac{aB}{B-b}\right)}{\left(\dfrac{aB}{B-b}\right) + C_A} = \frac{E_B B}{B + C_B}$$

which simplifies to

$$B = \frac{E_B C_A b + E_A a C_B}{a(E_B - E_A) + C_A E_B}. \tag{8.4}$$

Equation 8.4 applies to effects up to E_A. We call the dose of B that gives an effect $= E_A$ the critical value (Figure 8.1) which is given by

$$B_{crit} = \frac{E_A C_B}{E_B - E_A}. \tag{8.5}$$

For combination doses (a, b) in which b *is less than the critical value*, both drugs contribute to the effect, and this effect is found by calculating B from Equation 8.4 and using the calculated value in the dose-effect equation of drug B. As b approaches the critical value, the contribution of drug A becomes vanishingly small; that is, the relative potency $R = A/B$ increases without bound, and, thus, $b + a/R$ is entirely due to dose b of drug B. For values of b that are equal to or greater than the critical value, the effect is calculated as though drug B were acting alone.

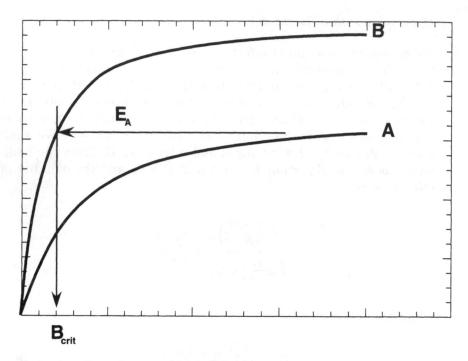

Figure 8.1. Dose-effect curves for two drugs with variable relative potency. The maximum effect of drug A corresponds to a dose of B denoted B_{crit}. Additive combinations (a, b) contribute to the effect when $b < B_{crit}$. When b equals or exceeds B_{crit} the additive effect is entirely due to dose b if the actions of the pair are independent.

Here it is important to recall the concept of independent joint action (Chapter 1) of the two drugs, the premise on which the above calculations are made. If the actions were not independent, say because each competes for a common cellular receptor, then these calculations would not apply. In that case, the dose of A, the partial agonist, would continue to contribute to the effect. If dose a became very large, it would dominate by displacing B molecules from the receptor. The result would be the maximum effect of drug A. This kind of interaction was termed "competitive dualism" by Ariens (1964). In the absence of mechanistic information *a priori*, the results of this kind of quantitative analysis are quite helpful in illuminating the mechanisms. For example, if experiments showed that A's contribution did vanish for doses b above the critical value, they would tend to confirm independent action. In contrast, if A's maximum effect is achieved when its dose is very large and b is somewhat above the critical value, then it would reveal itself as a sub-additive interaction in our classification scheme. This example illustrates how the quantitative approaches we have taken can contribute to understanding mechanism.

Nonparallel regression lines

We have seen from numerous examples that dose-effect data are often expressed by transforming to log dose and modeling the relation with linear regression analysis. If the regression lines are not parallel, the relative potency will change with the effect level. Usually regression lines of effect on log dose apply to effects that are not too near zero or 100% of the maximum effect. Therefore, the following analysis and illustration should be viewed with this restriction in mind. We shall denote the linear regression equation of drug A with parameters having subscript 1 and the equation of drug B with subscripts 2. The intercepts of each are then a_1 and a_2 and the regression coefficients (slopes) are b_1 and b_2. Thus,

Drug A: $$E = a_1 + b_1 \log A \qquad (8.6)$$

Drug B: $$E = a_2 + b_2 \log B. \qquad (8.7)$$

In this illustration it is assumed that these equations have been determined from the data for the individual drugs. If the analysis is based on probits, then E denotes the probit value (which is easily converted to a proportion from Table A.8 of the appendix). The additivity relation for the dose pair (a, b) is $a/A + b/B = 1$. To find the additive effect of this combination we equate the right hand sides of Equations 8.6 and 8.7 and solve simultaneously with the additive relation. Elimination of B from the additive relation leads to

$$c + b_1 \log A - b_2 \log A + b_2 \log (A - a) = 0 \qquad (8.8)$$

where $c = a_1 - a_2 - b_2 \log b$.

The value of A obtained as the solution of Equation 8.8 is used in Equation 8.6 to give the effect E of the combination. In other words, we have referred to the dose-effect curve of drug A. Had we eliminated A from the additivity condition, then a relation corresponding to Equation 8.8 would have B as the variable. In that case, the value of B obtained from the solution of the equation would be used in Equation 8.7 to get the additive effect.

The solution of Equation 8.8 cannot be obtained by algebraic methods. An iterative method (Newton-Raphson Method; see Tallarida, 1999) will give the solution to the desired degree of precision. This is accomplished by making an *initial estimate* of A, denoted A_0, and then calculating expression 8.8 at $A = A_0$ and the derivative at $A = A_0$. These are here denoted $f(A_0)$ and $f'(A_0)$, respectively, and are given by

$$f(A_0) = c + (0.4343)b_1 \ln A_0 - (0.4343)b_2 \ln A_0 \\ + (0.4343)b_2 \ln(A_0 - a) \tag{8.9}$$

and

$$f'(A_0) = 0.4343[b_1/A_0 - b_2/A_0 + b_2/(A_0 - a)]. \tag{8.10}$$

From these values an improved estimate is A_1 given by

$$A_1 = A_0 - \frac{f(A_0)}{f'(A_0)}. \tag{8.11}$$

The value of A_1 is next used as the estimate A_0 in Equations 8.9 and 8.10 which gives another A_1, etc. The process is continued until the absolute value of the difference between successive iterates is less than some designated small number, such as 0.01, meaning that no further improvement is needed.

Example. The regression lines shown in Figure 8.2 have values: $a_1 = -49$, $b_1 = 50$; $a_2 = 5$, and $b_2 = 67.96$. It was desired to determine the additive effect of the combination $a = 125$ and $b = 2$. The iterative procedure began with $A_0 = 150$. (Note from Equation 8.9 that A_0 must be greater than a). Iteration led to $A = 173.70$ and $B = 7.1333$ from which the effect is 62.99. Thus, the combination (125, 2) is expected to yield the effect 62.99. As a further confirmation of this additivity, note that $125/173.70 + 2/7.1333 = 1$.

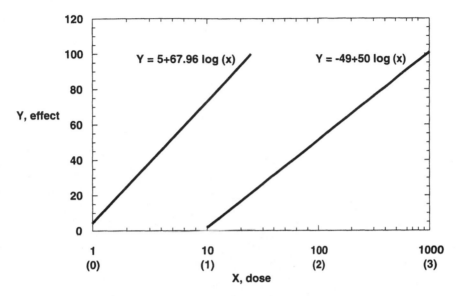

Figure 8.2. Regression lines for drug A and drug B. Values in parentheses along dose axis are logarithms of the doses (arbitrary units).

Figure 8.2

CHAPTER 8

References

Ariens, E.J. *Molecular Pharmacology* I. Acad. Press, N.Y., p. 169, 1964.
Tallarida, R.J. *Pocket Book of Integrals and Mathematical Formulas* 3rd ed. Chapman & Hall/CRC, Boca Raton, p. 68, 1999.

Different Experimental Designs

9.1   Combinations of an active and an inactive drug

Situations sometimes arise in which one of the two drugs of interest lacks efficacy or has very minor efficacy in the production of some effect. This chapter considers this type of combination. A combination of the agents is to be tested and, unless the inactive drug is a known competitive inhibitor, it is desired to know whether the combination of the two is additive or nonadditive. Sometimes the presence of the inactive drug produces an exaggerated effect. This situation occurs, for example, with [Leu⁵]enkephalin, a compound that shows no significant antinociception when administered by the intraperitoneal route in mice, but co-administration of morphine and [Leu⁵]enkephalin produces exaggerated antinociception as shown by Porreca et al. (1990). Our interest here is in quantitating such findings and demonstrating synergism.

For a fixed ratio combination of two agents A and B, we again denote by ρ_A the proportion that is drug A; hence, $1 - \rho_A$ is the proportion that is drug B in the combination. We will take drug B to be the inactive drug. Some level of effect, such as 50% of the maximum, is selected and we wish to compare the total amount of the combination that gives this effect with the calculated additive amount. These amounts will usually be concentrations or doses expressed as mg per kg of body weight. We denote the potency (e.g., D_{50} for 50% effect) of drug A by A. Then it is seen that the *total amount* in an additive combination is Z_{add} given by

$$Z_{add} = \frac{A}{\rho_A}.$$
(9.1)

The reasoning behind Equation 9.1 is straightforward. Since only drug A contributes to the effect, it is expected that the additive **total** must be greater than its own D_{50}. For example, if A represented only 1/3 of the total combination then the additive total should be three times its own D_{50} because of the dilution brought about by the presence of drug B.

Because A has a standard error, Z_{add} will have a standard error and this is given by

$$SE(Z_{add}) = \frac{SE(A)}{\rho_A}. \tag{9.2}$$

The quantity calculated from Equation 9.1 must be compared with the combination's D_{50}, denoted here by Z_{mix}. Synergism requires that $Z_{mix} < Z_{add}$, and thus the difference between these is used in a statistical test of the difference. (Usually the t-test is applied to the logarithms of Z_{add} and Z_{mix}.) In the [Leu⁵]enkephalin-morphine test, the estimate of A (the D_{50} of morphine) was obtained from regression of effect on log dose so that $A = 10^{\log A}$ and the standard error was calculated as $SE(A) = (2.30)(A)SE(\log A)$ (see Equation 2.12). A similar procedure was used to get Z_{mix} and its standard error from the combination regression of effect on log (total dose). Several fixed-ratio combinations of morphine and [Leu⁵]enkephalin were tested, and all showed synergism. The extent of the synergism is shown by the additive and mixture totals in Table 9.1.

The degree of synergism varied with the mixture ratio, being greatest for the 1:7 mixture.

Table 9.1. Values of Z_{add} and Z_{mix} (with S.E.M.) for Combinations of [Leu⁵]enkephalin and Morphine Sulfate. Combination Ratio (L:M) is Based on the Mass of the Constituents

Ratio	Z_{mix}	Z_{add}
1:3	13.9 (0.96)	20.5 (1.6)
1:5	18.9 (1.3)	30.7 (2.5)
1:6	16.4 (1.0)	35.8 (2.9)
1:7	10.9 (0.96)	41.0 (3.3)

Porreca et al., 1990.

9.2   Site-site interactions

Thus far our discussion of interactions has focused on combinations of two or more drugs and the combined effect of these. It is interesting to note that the mathematical formalism extends to *dual site* administration of the same compound. If, say, a drug is administered in the brain (intracerebroventricular, or i.c.v.) and simultaneously to another site, say the spinal cord (intrathecal, or i.th.), the combination will sometimes produce exaggerated effects. A well-known example of this *site-site interaction* is presented in the work of Yeung and Rudy (1980) which showed synergism when morphine was administered at the two sites.

Two-site administration has yielded other interesting results. Roerig et al. (1991) studied analgesic interactions with dual-site administration of either fentanyl, D-Ala^2-D-Leu^5 enkephalin (DADLE) or morphine in mice. They used i.c.v. and i.th. quantities of fentanyl (a *mu* opioid agonist) in normal mice and found additivity using an isobolographic analysis. But, when the same experiment was conducted in morphine-tolerant mice, the interaction became sub-additive. A quite different result emerged when the *delta* agonist DADLE was given to both sites in control and morphine-tolerant mice. This agonist showed simple site-site additivity in control animals and synergism in morphine-tolerant animals. These investigators further showed that morphine, given i.c.v. along with either i.th. fentanyl or DADLE in control animals, was synergistic. These studies have been useful in illuminating mechanisms and the role of receptor subtypes. (See the cited work for a detailed discussion and mechanistic interpretation.)

Acetaminophen in Two-Site Analysis

Acetaminophen is one of the most widely used analgesics, yet its mechanism is largely unknown. Many studies, using virtually every route of administration and many different animal antinociceptive tests, have not produced an understanding of the mechanism of this analgesic that was synthesized a century ago. (See discussion by Walker, 1995). Some evidence points to the central nervous system as the site of action (Bjorkman, 1995), but no clear mechanism has emerged. In an effort to approach the mechanistic question in a different way, Raffa et al. (1999) conducted experiments in which acetaminophen was injected either into the brain (i.c.v.) or into the spinal cord (i.th.) and, subsequently, into both sites simultaneously. The study was conducted in male mice and employed the abdominal irritant test described by Collier et al. (1968). Injections made by the i.c.v. route were to the right lateral cerebral ventricle (Haley and McCormick, 1957) whereas those injected i.th. were into the subarachnoid space by direct puncture of the subvertebral space between L5 and L6 (Hylden and Wilcox, 1980).

The i.c.v. injections produced no measurable antinociceptive effect, even for doses up to 1 μmole. In contrast, the intrathecal route produced clear dose-dependent antinociception. Assessment of effect was based on protection from an irritant injection during an observation period following its administration. Thus, the data collected were of the "all-or-none" variety. The results are given in Table 9.2. Because the i.c.v. route showed no effect, the calculation of the additive *ED50* (using probit analysis) is based on the i.th. data and the proportion of the total combination that was given this way; in this case, equal amounts were used.

As seen in Table 9.2, the *ED50* = 137 ± 22.6 μg, and the proportion, based on mass, is 0.5. Thus, from Equation 9.1, the calculated additive *ED50* = 274 ± 45. The actual combinations tested, shown in the table, gave *ED50* = 57.5 ± 8.55, a value significantly less than the additive estimate and, thus, indicative of marked synergism. The analysis leading to this result employs both design features discussed in this section: (1) one of the pair lacks efficacy and (2) site-site analysis. The result of this study is termed "self synergy," and it seems to be due to acetaminophen-induced release of a second substance from the brain that enters the cord to interact with acetaminophen at that site. Further studies aimed at identifying the released substance were underway at the time of this writing.

Table 9.2. Acetaminophen Given at Two Sites

i.th. (μg)	No. protected	No. tested	
45.35	5	50	
90.70	7	20	
151.17	11	18	
226.76	6	10	log (*ED50*) = 2.14 ± 0.072
			ED50 = 137 ± 22.6
i.th., i.c.v.			
11.34, 11.34	2	10	
22.68, 22.68	14	30	
45.35, 45.35	23	40	
90.70, 90.70	19	20	
			log(*ED50*) = 1.76 ± 0.065
			ED50 = 57.5 ± 8.55
Calculated additive values:			log (*ED50*) = 2.44 ± 0.072
			ED50 = 274 ± 45.

Site-Site Analysis with Opioid Receptor Subtypes

As a further indication of how combination analysis may illuminate mechanism, we point to experiments with δ_1 and δ_2-opioid agonists that were conducted in Hammond's laboratory (Hurley et al., 1999). These experiments were conducted in order to determine how delta-opioid receptor subtypes in the ventromedial medulla and the spinal cord interact to produce antinociception. To accomplish this, a single agent, either DPDPE (δ_1 type) or deltorphin (δ_2 type), was administered at both sites. Analysis of these experiments (tail-flick) revealed that concomitant administration of the δ_1 agonist, DPDPE resulted in a simply additive interaction. In contrast, the same procedure with the δ_2 agonist, deltorphin, produced a marked synergism. In fact, deltorphin at the two different sites appeared to be about 400 times more potent than the additive-predicted value. It was also found that at higher doses of deltorphin, the synergistic interaction converted to simple additivity, suggesting that different mechanisms mediate the antinociceptive effects of high and low doses of δ_2 agonists. These findings point out the role of receptor subtypes and suggest that synergistic interactions may result from receptor subtypes.

9.3   Theory of competitive antagonism

The main discussion thus far has been concerned with combinations of agonist compounds. Earlier in this chapter we considered the case of two compounds in which one of these showed little or no efficacy in the production of *a particular effect* according to the animal model tested. We now consider a situation in which one of the two drugs lacks efficacy and is actually known to be a competitive antagonist (*competitive inhibitor* is also used to describe such compounds). The earliest quantitative work in pharmacology aimed at receptor identification employed competitive antagonists in experiments with various agonists. We now consider this theory and its use.

When a fixed dose of a competitive antagonist is used in an experiment with graded doses of an agonist, it is possible to determine the affinity of the antagonist for the common receptor. This estimate of affinity provides a quantitative characterization of the receptor or receptor subtype. The theoretical basis for this kind of study is the *law of mass action* applied to the two competing agents. The agents, denoted A and B, each interact reversibly with receptor R, forming complexes AR and BR, respectively:

$$A + R \Leftrightarrow AR$$

$$B + R \Leftrightarrow BR.$$

At any time t we denote the concentration of AR by x and that of BR by y. The rate of formation of each is given by

$$\frac{dx}{dt} = k_{1A}A(R - x - y) - k_{2A}x \tag{9.3}$$

$$\frac{dy}{dt} = k_{1B}B(R - x - y) - k_{2B}y \tag{9.4}$$

where A, B, and R are the concentrations of compound A, compound B, and receptor, respectively, and the k's are forward and reverse rate constants that characterize each molecule's reaction with the common receptor. At equilibrium, the derivatives are both zero and thus the equilibrium concentrations x and y are given by

$$x_e = \frac{AR}{A + K_A\left(1 + \dfrac{B}{K_B}\right)} \tag{9.5}$$

and

$$y_e = \frac{BR}{B + K_B\left(1 + \dfrac{A}{K_A}\right)} \tag{9.6}$$

where K_A is k_{2A}/k_{1A} and K_B is k_{2B}/k_{1B}.

It is seen that each compound's binding is reduced because of the presence of the competing compound. If A is the active drug and B is an inactive drug, the biological effect will depend on the concentration x_e of A that is bound. It follows that the presence of B reduces the binding of A to the receptor and therefore reduces the effect. One need not make any assumption regarding the relation between effect and x_e (that is, no particular function is assumed to relate effect and occupancy), yet it is possible to obtain K_B from this theory and an experiment that produces dose-effect data.

Schild analysis

The experiment described here is one in which a fixed concentration of inhibitor B is used and dose-response data of A, in the presence of B, are obtained. The presence of B shifts the dose-effect curve to the right (Figure 9.1). At any level of effect, the concentrations of A are denoted by A in the absence of the competitor and A' in the presence of the competitor. These are equally effective concentrations and, therefore, x_e is the same in both situations. We therefore apply Equation 9.5 in the absence of B and in the presence of B and equate them:

$$\frac{AR}{A + K_A} = \frac{A'R}{A' + K_A\left(1 + \dfrac{B}{K_B}\right)}.$$

The above may be transformed to

$$\frac{A'}{A} - 1 = \frac{B}{K_B} \tag{9.7}$$

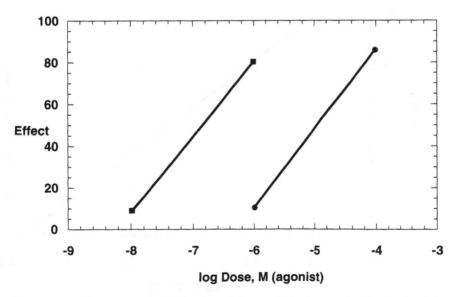

Figure 9.1. The line on the left is that of the agonist, whereas the line on the right is the agonist's dose-response relation in the presence of a fixed antagonist dose.

which is equivalent to

$$\log\left(\frac{A'}{A} - 1\right) = -(-\log B) - \log K_B. \tag{9.8}$$

For the known concentration B and the experimentally determined ratio (A'/A), either of the above equations allows a calculation of K_B. A common procedure is to use the logarithmic form in a plot that uses several different values of B and the experimentally produced agonist dose ratios. This plot, called a *Schild plot* as shown in Figure 9.2, is theoretically a straight line with slope $= -1$ and intercept $-\log K_B$. The intercept is therefore an indicator of the logarithm of $1/K_B$. If the actual data produced a plot with slope $= -1$, both intercepts would be the same, and, thus, each gives the value of K_B. In practice, the slope (usually determined from linear regression) is not exactly -1. If the slope does not differ significantly from -1, this will usually mean that the data are acceptable and that the departure from unit slope is due to uncertainty

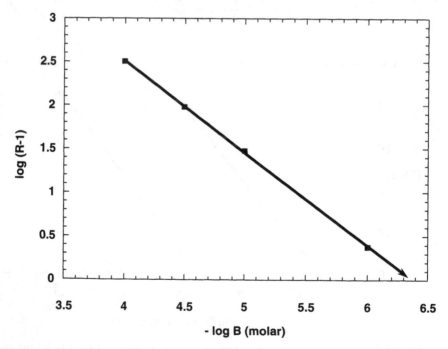

Figure 9.2. Schild plot for the data in Table 9.3. The pA_2 value is indicated by the arrow; for these data, $pA_2 = 6.37 \pm 0.025$. In this plot $-\log B$ is used, thereby producing slope $= -1$.

(scatter) in the data. In practice, one takes the horizontal intercept which was called pA_2 by Schild (Arunlakshana and Schild, 1959) when concentration B is in molar units.

Because this intercept is derived from a plot that has scatter, the confidence limits of the intercept are reported along with the pA_2 value. When the slope does not differ significantly from −1, the pA_2 is related to a fundamental receptor constant (K_B). When the slope departs from −1, the pA_2 is merely a measure of the degree of antagonism. Values of K_B determined from Schild plots have been used to characterize receptors and receptor subtypes. Examples of this kind of analysis are numerous and the topic has been reviewed (Tallarida et al., 1979). A more recent application, concerned with inhibition of platelet aggregation, is described by Vezza et al. (1997). An example of Schild analysis is provided below.

Example. *Schild Analysis.* Four doses of a competitive antagonist produced shifts in the agonist dose-response curve that were expressed as the agonist dose ratio $R = (A'/A)$. The data (simulated for illustration) are shown in Table 9.3. The data in the table were analyzed with linear regression (Chapter 2) and Equation 2.9 was applied to get the standard error of the pA_2 that is given in the legend of Figure 9.2.

Table 9.3. Each Antagonist Dose (*B*) Produces a Dose Ratio (Shift) *R*

B	−log (B)	R − 1	log (R − 1)
10^{-4}	4.0000	320	2.50
3.16×10^{-5}	4.5003	97	1.99
10^{-5}	5.0000	30	1.48
10^{-6}	6.0000	2.4	0.38

9.4   Combined inhibitory effects

Having discussed competitive inhibition in a book that is mainly concerned with the combined action of agonist agents, we felt it reasonable to ask whether *two inhibitors* ever show synergism. Braverman and Ruggieri (2000) conducted this kind of experiment with muscarinic agents that affect the bladder (in rat). The bladder was surgically denervated and, following a three-day recovery period, was excised and cut into strips for testing tension development in response to carbachol. At a level of carbachol that produced a desired effect level (% of maximum), one or the other of two competitive inhibitors were added in varying doses (ng/ml). These were methoctramine-tetrahy-drochloride (Meth) and parafluorohexahydrosila-diphenadol HCl (pf). Each produced a diminution of the tension, thereby indicating receptor blockade. A 10:1 combination (based on mass) of the inhibitors was subsequently used. Table 9.4 shows the data from a preliminary experiment and a detailed regression analysis that includes the D_{50} values for each inhibitor, the additive D_{50}, and the actual (mixture) D_{50}. (The D_{50} for inhibition is often denoted IC_{50}). Because the mixture D_{50} is significantly less than the additive D_{50}, the combination of inhibitors in the fixed ratio used ($\rho = 0.9091$) is synergistic. This finding may be due to the fact that these are not entirely receptor-specific antagonists; that is, each is only relatively selective for a specific muscarinic receptor. In that case their actions are not independent (see Chapter 1) and, therefore, some interaction would be expected. However, the same experiment carried out in normal animals (i.e., not denervated) produced results that showed simple additivity (data not given here). Thus, the nature of the interaction is not yet understood, and the problem is undergoing further study at the time of this writing.

Table 9.4. Combination of Inhibitors of Carbachol in the Rat Bladder

	Data Set: Denervated: Meth	
Dose[1]	Log(dose)	Effect[2]
457.7	2.661	12.6
1405.7	3.148	19.7
4537	3.657	38.2
13840.2	4.141	63.6

Eqn: $Y = 34.64x - 84.30$ $r = 0.972$
  slope $= 34.64 \pm 2.94$
    $\bar{x} = 3.401$ $S_{xx} = 1.225$
    $\bar{y} = 33.525$ $S_{xy} = 42.45$
                                              $s = 6.522$
  $SS_{tot} = 1555$
  $SS_{res} = 85.07$ $\log D_{50} = 3.877 \pm 0.124$
  $SS_{reg} = 1470$ $D_{50} = 7538 \pm 2152$

                                                        (*continued*)

[1]   ng/ml

[2]   % of maximum

Table 9.4. (Continued) Combination of Inhibitors of Carbachol in the Rat Bladder

Data Set: Denervated : Pf		
Dose	Log(dose)	Effect
138.8	2.142	24.3
457.7	2.661	32.8
1406	3.148	42.3
4537	3.657	64.9
13840	4.141	72

Eqn: $Y = = 25.53x -33.17$ $\qquad$ $r = 0.983$
  slope $= 25.53 \pm 1.245$
  $\bar{x} = 3.150$ $\qquad$ $S_{xx} = 2.494$
  $\bar{y} = 47.26$ $\qquad$ $S_{xy} = 63.68$
  $\qquad$ $s = 4.397$

$SS_{tot} = 1684$
$SS_{res} = 58.00$ $\qquad$ $\log D_{50} = 3.257 \pm 0.078$
$SS_{reg} = 1626$ $\qquad$ $D_{50} = 1807.4 \pm 324$

Composite Parameters $f = 0.7057$
$\rho_1 = 0.9091$
$Z_{add}(C) = 5745.2041 \pm 759.1420$

Data Set: Composite Additive		
Dose	Log(dose)	Effect
250.3	2.398	12.6
662.7	2.821	24.3
833.5	2.921	19.7
1940	3.288	32.8
3216	3.507	38.2
5158	3.712	42.3
11308	4.053	64.9
11692	4.068	63.6
30214	4.480	72

Eqn: $Y = 30.80x -65.81$ $\qquad$ $r = 0.977$
  slope $= 30.80 \pm 0.841$
  $\bar{x} = 3.472$ $\qquad$ $S_{xx} = 3.682$

(continued)

Table 9.4. (Continued) Combination of Inhibitors of Carbachol in the Rat Bladder

y – int = –65.80748 ± / –8.912029
$\bar{y}$ = 41.16 S_{xy} = 113.4
                                               s = 4.844
SS_{tot} = 3658
SS_{res} = 164.2   Log D_{50} = 3.75 ± 0.0574
SS_{reg} = 3494 D_{50} = 5745 ± 759

Data Set: Denervated Mix

Combination Parameters f = 0.7057
ρ_1 = 0.9091

Dose	Log(dose)	Effect
457.7	2.661	25.1
1406	3.148	38
4537	3.657	65.1
13840	4.141	86

Eqn: Y = 42.41x –90.71   r = 0.992
  slope = 42.41 ± 1.85
  $\bar{x}$ = 3.402 S_{xx} = 1.225
  $\bar{y}$ = 53.55 S_{xy} = 51.97
                                               s = 4.094
SS_{tot} = 2237.61
SS_{res} = 33.51831   log D_{50} = 3.318 ± 0.049
SS_{reg} = 2204.092 D_{50} = 2079.13 ± 233
Statistics: F = 16.53 t' = 5.855   T = 3.177

CHAPTER 9

References

Arunlakshana O. and Schild, H.O. Some quantitative use of drug antagonists. *Br. J. Pharmacol.* 14:48, 1959.

Braverman, A. and Ruggieri, M. Submitted for publication, 2000.

Bjorkman, R. *Acta Anaesthesiol. Scand.* 39 (Suppl. 103):2, 1995.

Collier, H.O., Dinneen, L.C., Johnson, C.A., and Schneider, C. The abdominal constriction response and its suppression by analgesic drugs in the mouse. *Brit. J. Pharmacol.* 32:295, 1968.

Haley, T.J. and McCormick, W.G. Pharmacological effects produced by intracerebral injections of drugs in the conscious mouse. *Brit. J. Pharmacol.* 12:12, 1957.

Hylden, J.L.K. and Wilcox, G.L. Intrathecal morphine in mice: a new technique. *Eur. J. Pharmacol.* 67: 313, 1980.

Hurley, R.W., Grabow, T.S., Tallarida, R.J., and Hammond, D.L. Interaction between medullary and spinal delta-1 and delta-2 opioid receptors in the production of antinociception in the rat. *J. Pharmacol. Exp. Ther.* 289:993–999, 1999.

Porreca, F., Jiang, Q., and Tallarida, R.J. Modulation of morphine antinociception by peripheral [Leu⁵]enkephalin: a synergistic interaction. *Eur. J. Pharmacol.*179:463–468, 1990

Raffa, R.B., Stone, D., and Tallarida, R.J. Abstract. Antinociceptive self synergy between spinal and supraspinal acetaminophen (paracetamol). *Int. Assoc. for the Study of Pain*, Austria, 1999.

Roerig, S.G., Hoffman, R.G., Takemori, A.E., Wilcox, G.L., and Fujimoto, J.M. Isobolographic analysis of analgesic interactions between intrathecally and intracerebroventricularly administered fentanyl, morphine and D-Ala²-D-Leu⁵ enkephalin in morphine-tolerant and nontolerant mice. *J. Pharmacol. Exp. Ther.* 257:1091–1099, 1991.

Tallarida, R.J., Cowan, A., and Adler, M.W. pA_2 and receptor differentiation: A statistical analysis of competitive antagonism. *Life Sci.* 25:637–653, 1979.

Vezza, R., Spina, D., Tallarida, R.J., Malevika, N., Page, C.P., and Gresele, P. Antivasoconstrictor and antiaggregatory activities of picotamide unrelated to thromboxane A2 antagonism. *Thromb. Haem.* 78:1385–91, 1997.

Walker, J.S. NSAID: an update on their analgesic effects. *Clin. Exper. Pharmacol. Physiol.* 22:855, 1995.

Yeung, J.C. and Rudy, R.A. Multiplicative interaction between narcotic agonisms expressed at spinal and supraspinal sites of action as revealed by
concurrent intrathecal and intracerebroventricular injections of morphine.
J. Pharmacol. Exp. Ther. 215:633–642, 1980.

CHAPTER 10

Response Surface Analysis
of Drug Combinations

Combinations of two drugs lead to effects that depend on the constituent doses. It may be desirable to produce a plot of the effect for each dose combination. This kind of plot and the procedures used to make and analyze it provide methodology for measuring the synergism at any particular dose combination and effect level. (This is in contrast to the isobole method that measures synergism at a single, specified effect level.) The dose of each drug is an independent variable and the effect is the dependent variable. A three-dimensional plot results. The doses are plotted on the plane in a three-dimensional Cartesian coordinate system as individual points. The effect of a dose pair is plotted as the vertical distance above the point. Since each dose of the pair defining the combination is a continuous variable, the dose pair points lie in a region over which there is a continuum of effects. The three-dimensional plot is therefore a surface. Each measured effect (response) is a point that defines this response surface.

If the data from each compound are fitted to a smooth curve, such as the common hyperbolic curve, the surface of an additive combination of doses is also smooth and is completely determinable. If actual combination doses produce effects that are greater than additive, then these points will be located above the additive surface. Each of these super-additive effects can be characterized by the value of the interaction index which measures the strength of the synergism for the dose pair.

10.1 Additive combinations and response surface

We are concerned here with a situation in which each of the two compounds (denoted A and B) produces a dose-dependent effect, i.e., each yields a dose-effect relation for the common effect being studied.

We denote these relations with functional notation, $E = f(A)$ for compound A, and $E = g(B)$ for compound B. As we have seen, the two compounds may produce either additive or nonadditive actions when they are given together as the dose combination (a, b). An additive action occurs when the constituents contribute to the effect in accordance with their individual potencies. For example, if drug A has twice the potency of drug B, then, in combination, A may be substituted for B in an amount that is one half the amount that would be required of B. By using the relative potency of the agents, the combination may be referred to either compound. For example, if A is the reference compound, then (a, b) may be expressed as an equivalent amount of A when it acts alone. For a simply additive interaction with relative potency R (= *dose A/dose B*) *the same at every level of effect*, the calculation of the dose of A that is equivalent to (a, b) is given by

$$A_{eq} = a + Rb. \tag{10.1}$$

Because the effect E for any dose of A is known (from its dose-effect curve, $E = f(A)$) the dose combination (a, b), that yields A_{eq} from the above equation can be paired with this effect by using the calculated A_{eq} in the relation, $E = f(A)$. A graphical view of this pairing is provided in a plot of E against (a, b), a procedure that yields a surface above the domain of (a, b) points. In other words, the pair (a, b) is a point in the plane, and the effect is plotted as the vertical distance above it (Figure 10.1). The response surface obtained this way (use of Equation 10.1) applies to simply additive combinations and is therefore an *additive response surface*. The procedure for getting the plot coordinates is illustrated in the following example in which the individual dose-effect curves have been constructed so that the relative potency is constant. Any dose pair (a, b) leads to an equivalent dose of A calculated from Equation 10.1. This equivalent dose A_{eq} is used in the relation, $E = f(A)$ to get the effect level E.

Example. Two compounds A and B have dose-effect relations shown in Figure 10.2. The relative potency is constant and found to be 2.32. The dose-effect equation of A, which we take as the reference compound, is given by the equation, $E = 100 \, A/(A + 11.24)$. From Equation 10.1, any pair of doses (a, b) is converted to an equivalent, $A_{eq} = (a + 2.32 \, b)$. When the value A_{eq}, calculated this way, is inserted into the dose-effect equation for compound A, we get the expected additive effect. For example, point $(1, 2)$ gives $A_{eq} = 1 + 2.32 \times 2 = 5.64$ and this dose of A gives

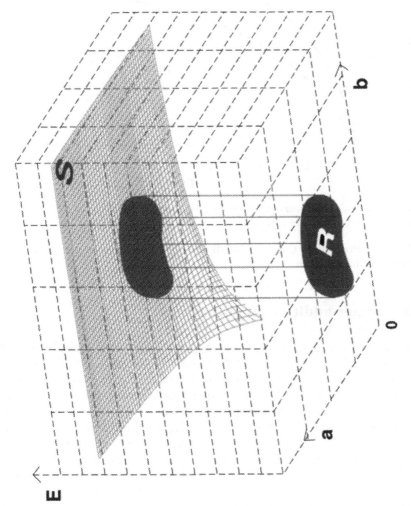

Figure 10.1. A dose pair (a,b) corresponds to a point in the plane, and the vertical distance above it indicates its effect. The totality of dose combinations would produce a surface (S) in this three-dimensional plot. Dose combinations contained within the shaded region (R) in the plane result in effects indicated by the corresponding region on the surface. (Courtesy of J. McCary.)

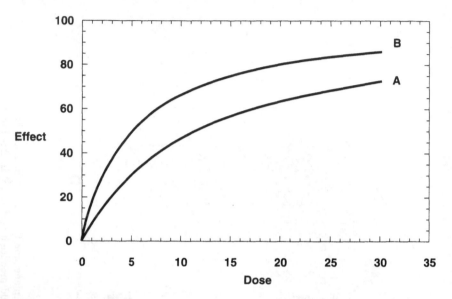

Figure 10.2. Dose-effect curves for compounds A and B. The relative potency is 2.32, compound B being the more potent.

$E = 33.4$. Proceeding this way for all dose combinations we get the additive response surface.

10.2   Super-additive combinations

When a dose combination is super-additive (synergistic) and the relative potency R is constant, the dose pair (a, b) acts like the greater dose $(a + R b)/\alpha$, where α, the *interaction index*, is less than unity. This relation follows from the simultaneous solution of $R = A/B$ and $a/A + b/B = \alpha$. This directly relates the additive equivalent to the dose corresponding to the observed effect of the combination. Stated differently, the interaction index is a mathematical factor (multiplier) that indicates the degree of dosage reduction in a combination in order to get the effect of A alone or B alone. With reference to compound A's dose-effect relation (curve) the greater dose, $(a + Rb)/\alpha$, produces a different (greater) effect than the additive effect. The three-dimensional plot of effect vs. (a, b) would therefore be a surface positioned above the additive response surface.

The interaction index is calculated from tests with combination (a, b). For such a pair, the effect is measured, and this value is related to the corresponding dose of A from its dose-effect relation (curve). That dose, A_{corr} is then used in the following equation

$$A_{corr} = (a + Rb)/\alpha = A_{eq}/\alpha. \qquad (10.2)$$

This equation allows a determination of α. In our previous example we saw that (1, 2) gave A_{eq} = 5.64 and the additive effect 33.4. Suppose, however, that the observed effect of this dose pair were 45 instead of 33.4. This magnitude of effect, 45, corresponds to dose A_{corr} = 9.20, a value that we obtain from the dose-effect equation for compound A. From Equation 10.2, we have 9.20 = 5.64/α; thus, α = 0.613. This procedure calculates the degree of synergism (expressed as the interaction index α) for all actual dose pairs tested. It should be noted that the relative potency R is an *estimated* quantity as are the dose-effect relations of the constituent drugs. For this reason several experiments with the same (*a*, *b*) combination should be conducted, thereby giving a set of values of the interaction index α. From these values a mean and standard error may be obtained. The calculation of α is straightforward because the relative potency (R) is a constant. We next discuss the calculation of α when R varies with the effect level.

10.3   Variable relative potency

When the relative potency varies with the effect level the individual dose-effect curves, $E_A = f(A)$ and $E_B = g(B)$, provide the values of R and, thus, A_{eq}. To get the *additive* equivalent of A in this situation the effects are equated, $f(A) = g(B)$, and this equation is solved simultaneously with the additive relation

$$a/A + b/B = 1. \qquad (10.3)$$

Equation 10.3 is the same as Equation 10.1 except that R (=A/B) is now a variable that does not appear explicitly. Its value depends on the functions f and g and, therefore, it is implicit in the solution of the simultaneous equations. The value of A determined from these simultaneous equations is A_{eq} and is obtained by eliminating B. The value of A_{eq} is used to calculate the effect level from drug A's dose-effect equation (curve) as previously described. This calculated effect level is the expected effect for pair (*a*, *b*) under additivity and a plot of these gives the additive response surface. Whether the relative potency is constant or variable, it is seen that the additive surface is completely determined from the individual dose-effect curves. *Synergism in this situation of varying R, described by a/A + b/B = α, is not characterized by a simple relation such as Equation 10.2.* Instead, a new relation is derived in the following way. The effect of (a, b) is determined by testing, and this effect is referred to drug A's dose-effect equation (curve) in order to get the corresponding dose, A_{corr}. Simultaneous solution of the equations, $a/A + b/B = α$ and $f(A) = g(B)$, eliminates B and gives the relation between $α$ and $A(=A_{corr})$, thereby providing the value of $α$ for the dose pair. The following example illustrates the calculation.

Table 10.1. Dose-Effect Data with Variable R

A		B	
Dose	Effect	Dose	Effect
0	0	0	0
10	32	4	40
15	40	6	50
30	53	10	62
45	60	20	76
		30	83
		45	88

Example. The data sets below were made up to illustrate the situation in which two compounds have a varying potency ratio. The values of dose and effect (arbitrary units) are given in Table 10.1 for compounds A and B:

These data sets are well described by the equations

$$E_A = \frac{80A}{A + 15} \quad \text{and} \quad E_B = \frac{100B}{B + 6}.$$

We now consider the system of equations:

$$\frac{80A}{A + 15} = \frac{100B}{B + 6} \quad \text{and} \quad \frac{a}{A} + \frac{b}{B} = α.$$

Elimination of B gives the following relation that relates the doses a, b and $α$ to the A corresponding to the observed effect:

$$24a + 75b + bA - 24αA = 0$$

Now suppose that testing with doses $a = 2$, $b = 3$, produces an effect = 60. From the dose-effect relation of compound A, an effect = 60 means that dose $A = 45$. Substitution of $a = 2$, $b = 3$, and $A = 45$ in the above yields $\alpha = 0.378$. In this same way the interaction index is determinable for all combinations tested. Of course, only effects that are achieved by both compounds can be used in this analysis.

Dose-effect relations

The previous analysis shows that whether the relative potency of the two compounds is constant or variable over the range of effects, it is still possible to determine the value of α from the combination data and thereby distinguish additivity from super-additivity. This analysis requires suitable equations for modeling each compound's dose-effect relation. The (graded) dose-effect relation of a drug has been modeled in a number of ways; a common model is the hyperbolic relation used in the previous example and given by $E = E_{max}(D)/[(D) + C]$. In this equation the constant C is equivalent to the dose (D) that gives the half-maximal effect (D_{50} dose). If each drug also produces the same maximum effect, then R, the relative potency, determined from the hyperbolic relation is a constant equal to the ratio of the C's of each agent: $R = C_A/C_B$. (Other nonlinear models are discussed in Chapter 11.) Another common model is the linear log(dose)-effect relation. When the two linear relations give parallel lines, the relative potency is constant whereas nonparallel lines mean a varying R. Whether R is a constant or a variable, the parameter α can be determined as we just showed. It should be recalled that the dose-effect curves of the individual drugs allow one to calculate the additive total dose, Z_{add}, for a specified effect level (isobole method described in Chapter 4). The value of Z_{add} is then compared to the total dose of the combination (Z_{mix}) that gives the same effect experimentally. A synergistic interaction gives a total dose Z_{mix} that is equal to $\alpha\, Z_{add}$.

10.4   Response surface analysis of morphine and clonidine

There have been several quantitative studies of the combination of spinal morphine and clonidine (Wilcox et al., 1987; Ossipov et al., 1990, 1990a; Fairbanks and Wilcox, 1999), including a study we conducted (Tallarida et al., 1997). One aspect of these was discussed in Chapter

4, in which we illustrated the isobole method for effect level = 50% of the maximum. That analysis used linear regression of effect on log dose as the model and employed one fixed-ratio combination. That fixed dose ratio revealed synergism and was a confirmation of earlier work by Ossipov et al. (1990; 1990a) who found synergism when the drugs were administered intrathecally. It was desired to examine this combination in a response surface analysis that employed other fixed ratio combinations (Tallarida et al., 1999). In this study, the mouse tail immersion test was used with hot water (55°C) as the nociceptive stimulus using the protocol described by Raffa and Stone (1996). Intrathecal administration via injection into the subvertebral space between L5 an L6 (Hylden and Wilcox, 1980) was employed. Antinociception was measured as an increase in tail-withdrawal latency and was converted to percent of maximum percent effect (*MPE*) according to the formula: %*MPE* = 100 × (test latency − control latency)/(15 − control latency). The 15-s cutoff was used to avoid injury to the tail. For construction of the dose-effect curves the effect was expressed as mean %*MPE*, from 10 mice per dose, and was assessed at the time of peak effect (10 min after drug administration).

Morphine-clonidine data

The combination experiment produced data that are continuous on the effect scale and are shown in Table 10.3. But first we must examine the dose-effect data for each drug, used alone, in Table 10.2. These data allow a calculation of the additive total dose for each fixed ratio combination which may then be compared statistically to the actual total dose for the same fixed ratio combination in order to distinguish syn-

Table 10.2. Dose-Effect Data[a]

Morphine SO$_4$		Clonidine HCl	
Dose	Effect	Dose	Effect
1.138	19.67	0.800	19.79
3.793	40.32	2.667	31.40
11.38	61.91	7.998	74.92
37.93	88.52	26.66	92.41
$D_{50} = 5.856 \pm 0.52$		$D_{50} = 3.787 \pm 0.78$	

[a] Dose of the salt (μg) and effect as mean% *MPE* based on 10 animals and use of the hyperbolic model in which the constant $C = D_{50}$.

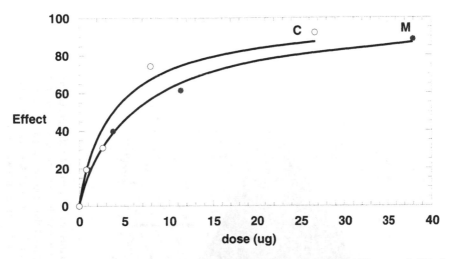

Figure 10.3. The dose-response data for morphine (M) and clonidine (C) are each fitted to a hyperbolic model from which the relative potency is 1.546.

ergism from simple additivity. That kind of analysis (use of total dose), previously made for one combination of these agents, was illustrated in Chapter 4. The objective in this chapter is to present the data for two additional combinations and, in so doing, utilize the response surface approach that uses the dose pairs as previously described.

Each drug's dose-effect data were fitted to the hyperbolic relation, $E = E_{max}(D)/[(D) + C]$ over the range of effects, 0 to 100 = E_{max}. (In Chapter 4 these data sets were modeled with linear regression.) Correlation coefficients, 0.993 for the morphine curve and 0.975 for the clonidine curve confirm the good fits (Figure 10.3). The constant C (= D_{50}) for each is given in Table 10.2. As previously noted, this kind of fit means that the potency ratio R is also a constant = C_A/C_B = 1.546 in this case. It is thus possible to construct the additive response surface for these drugs in a three-dimensional plot (Figure 10.4). The additive equation is given by

$$E = \frac{E_{max}(a + Rb)}{(a + Rb) + C_A}.$$ (10.4)

The super-additive equation, for constant α, is given by

$$E = \frac{E_{max}(a + Rb)/\alpha}{(a + Rb)/\alpha + C_A}.$$ (10.5)

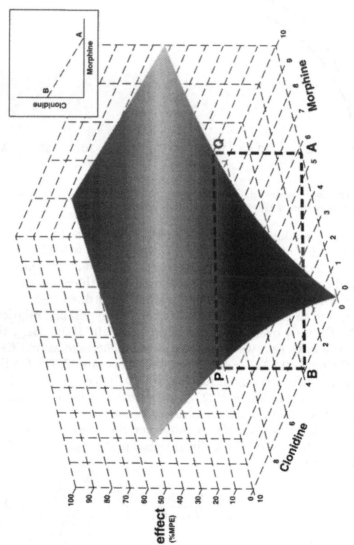

Figure 10.4. The additive response surface is a smooth convex surface. On this surface a contour of equal effects gives the projection in the dose plane that is the familiar additive isobole, a line with intercepts *A* and *B* on the dose axes. In contrast, a super-additive surface would have a projection that is off the additive line and contained within the region formed by the line and the axes. The amount by which this trace is off the line is a visual indicator of the degree of synergism but is not obviously represented on the isobologram in a way that shows its precise measure. (From Tallarida, R.J., Stone, D.J., McCary, J.D., and Raffa, R.B. A response surface analysis of synergism between morphine and clonidine. *J. Pharmacol. Exp. Ther.* 289:8–13, 1999. Used with permission.)

The amount of surface elevation for a synergistic dose (a, b) can be determined from the above equations as the difference of the E's.

Before examining the results of the combination experiments, it is instructive to view the response surface for a synergistic (super-additive) interaction of these drugs. To accomplish this illustration we have constructed such a surface using $\alpha = 0.1$ (Figure 10.5). This is an illustrative example in which a value of α indicative of strong (but realistic) synergism is used (as will be shown subsequently); moreover, this illustration includes the assumption of a single value of α that characterizes the drug combination. This assumption was examined in the current study by calculating the values of α for all dose pairs tested and is described subsequently, but the graph of Figure 10.5, based on a single value of α, is nevertheless revealing. It shows a uniformly smooth response surface, convex and clearly positioned above the simply additive surface. The extent to which a single value of α and with this magnitude (0.1), applies to the current data is revealed in an analysis of the actual combination data obtained.

The data shown in Table 10.3 provide the results of the combination experiments along with the calculated additive equivalent of drug A (morphine) as well as the amount of A (A_{corr}) that corresponds to the actual combination effect observed. Three different sets of fixed ratio combinations were used. In the first set, the proportion of morphine SO_4 was 0.605, while in sets 2 and 3 the proportions were 0.338 and 0.821, respectively. For each drug combination, the parameter α was calculated by relating the observed effect to get A_{corr}, calculating A_{eq} and applying Equation 10.2 as previously described. These values are given in the table. It is seen from the values of α that there is marked synergism. But the actual α values show a difference for each combination set tested. To test whether the mean value of this interaction index differs among the three dose sets, we examined the groups in an analysis of variance followed by the Newman Keuls test (described in Chapter 12). The result, shown in Table 10.4, indicates significance, $p < 0.05$. These statistical results indicate that the mean value of α for set 1 is greater than the values for the other two sets which do not differ significantly. In other words, there is synergism for each of the three dose proportions tested, but the synergism is more pronounced in sets 2 and 3 than in set 1.

10.5   Isobolar analysis or surface analysis

The values of the interaction index α shown in Table 10.3 were determined from each combination's observed effect, the values of A_{corr} and

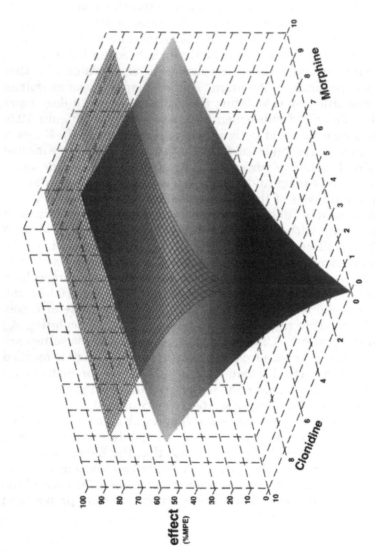

Figure 10.5. A super-additive surface for a constant value of the interaction index = 0.1 is positioned above the additive surface. Actual data showed that the interaction index for morphine + clonidine was not constant over the surface but had mean values of 0.303, 0.101, and 0.051 for the three fixed ratio combinations tested. (From Tallarida, R.J., Stone, D.J., McCary, J.D., and Raffa, R.B. A response surface analysis of synergism between morphine and clonidine. *J. Pharmacol. Exp. Ther.* 289:8–13, 1999. Used with permission.)

Table 10.3. Combination Dose-Effect Data and Calculated Quantities for Morphine and Clonidine in Three Different Fixed Ratio Combinations

Comb.	Doses (a, b)* (μg)	Effect	A_{eq}	A_{corr}	α
Set 1	0.360, 0.235	20.21	0.723	1.483	0.487
	0.720, 0.470	38.96	1.447	3.738	0.387
	1.44, 0.940	65.98	2.893	11.357	0.255
	2.88, 1.88	92.04	5.786	67.71	0.085
				mean	**0.303**
Set 2	0.0225, 0.044	28.42	0.0905	2.325	0.039
	0.045, 0.088	35.58	0.181	3.234	0.056
	0.090, 0.176	42.96	0.362	4.410	0.082
	0.180, 0.352	81.26	0.724	25.39	0.029
	0.719, 1.408	90.81	2.896	57.86	0.050
				mean	**0.051**
Set 3	0.1347, 0.0292	14.4	0.1799	0.985	0.183
	0.269, 0.0585	47.66	0.3599	5.332	0.0675
	0.539, 0.117	69.50	0.7199	13.34	0.0539
	1.079, 0.235	69.45	1.442	13.31	0.1083
				mean	**0.101**

* Dose (a, b) is (morphine.SO_4, clonidine.HCl) per mouse. Each effect is the mean from at least 10 observations.

Table 10.4. Analysis of Variance of Interaction Index (α) for Different Fixed Ratio Combinations

Source of variation	Sum of squares	D.F	Mean square	F
Total	0.2539	12		
Between	0.1517	2	0.0758	7.42
Within	0.1022	10	0.0102	

the additive equivalent dose, A_{eq}, of reference drug A (morphine) calculated from Equation 10.1. The data for these three sets, however, also permit estimations of α based on the 50% effect level. Toward this end we utilize the calculated additive total dose for %MPE = 50, denoted Z_{add}, and the total dose, Z_{mix}, that gives %MPE = 50. The value Z_{mix} was obtained by curve-fitting the total dose-effect data to the hyperbolic model, while Z_{add} is calculated from Equation 4.12. The values Z_{add} and Z_{mix} for the 50% effect level are shown in Table 10.5.

Table 10.5. Equieffective Total Doses and Interaction Index for %*MPE* = 50

Combination	Set 1	Set 2	Set 3
Proportion[a]	$\rho = 0.605$	$\rho = 0.338$	$\rho = 0.821$
Z_{add}	4.82	4.30	5.33
Z_{mix}	1.43	0.223	0.414
α	0.297	0.052	0.077

[a] The proportion of the total mass that is morphine sulfate. The proportions are based on estimated D_{50} values of the morphine (M) and clonidine (C) constituents: Set 1, 0.5 (M), 0.5 (C); Set 2, 0.25 (M), 0.75 (C); Set 3, 0.75 (M), 0.25 (C).

The ratio, Z_{mix}/Z_{add}, provides an estimation of α for the 50% level. The values of α determined this way are given in Table 10.5 for each of the three fixed ratio combination sets. This method of determining α used equieffective total doses, Z_{add} and Z_{mix}, and is therefore the isobole method we have previously used (Chapter 4) to test for synergism. These estimates of the interaction index for the three sets (Table 10.5) have the same order relation as the mean values of the index that were obtained from actual effects over the surface (Table 10.3).

The isobole method uses doses of the individual drugs and the drug combinations that produce some particular effect such as 50% of the maximum. In contrast, the response surface approach examines all tested combinations and the effects they produce, thereby obtaining values of the interaction index for each combination. This more detailed examination allows one to view the effects of both small and large dose combinations and, thus, determine if the nature of the interaction is dose dependent. This information may be useful in uncovering mechanism. (See, for example, Hurley et al., 1999; Meissler et al., 1998.) We saw, however, in the study just described, that the three different fixed ratio combinations produced mean values of α that had the same order relation as those obtained from the isobole method. The choice of method will be dictated by the purpose of the study. It should also be recalled that different tests can give different results. For example, in tests of antinociception, the nature of the nociceptive stimulus may affect the efficacy and the potency of the individual compounds and, thus, their combined effect. In other words, different neuronal mechanisms may underlie each stimulus and the modulatory role of the drugs on responses to the stimulus. A good example is provided in Adams et al. (1993).

CHAPTER 10

References

Adams, J.U., Tallarida, R.J., Geller, E.B., and Adler, M.W. Isobolographic superadditivity between delta and mu opioid agonists in the rat depends on the ratio of the compounds, the mu agonist and the analgesic assay used. *J. Pharmacol. Exp. Ther.* 266:1261–1267, 1993.

Fairbanks, C.A. and Wilcox, G.I. Spinal antinociceptive synergism between morphine and clonidine persists in mice made acutely or chronically tolerant to morphine. *J. Pharmacol. Exp. Ther.* 288:1107–1116, 1999.

Hurley, R.W., Grabow, T.S., Tallarida, R.J., and Hammond, D L. Interaction between medullary and spinal delta-1 and delta-2 opioid receptors in the production of antinociception in the rat. *J. Pharmacol. Exp. Ther.* 289:993–999, 1999.

Hylden, J.L.K. and Wilcox, G.L. Intrathecal morphine in mice: a new technique. *Eur. J. Pharmacol.* 67:313–316, 1980.

Meissler Jr., J.J., Adler, M.W., Rogers, T.J., Geller, E.B., Tallarida, R.J., and Eisenstein, T.K. Super- and sub-additive interactions of morphine and deltorphin in inducing immunosuppression. NIDA Monograph Series. 178:200, 1998.

Ossipov, M.H., Harris, S., Lloyd, P., and Messineo, E. An isobolographic analysis of the antinociceptive effect of systemically and intrathecally administered combinations of morphine and clonidine. *J. Pharmacol. Exp. Ther.* 255:1107–1115, 1990.

Ossipov, M.H., Lozito, R., Messineo, E., Green, J., Harris. S., and Lloyd, P. Spinal antinociceptive synergy between clonidine and morphine, U69593, and DPDPE: Isobolographic analysis. *Life Sci.* 46:PL71–PL76, 1990a.

Raffa, R.B. and Stone, D.J. Could dual G-protein coupling explain [D-Met2]-FMRFamide's mixed action in vivo? *Peptides* 17:1261–1265, 1996.

Tallarida, R.J., Stone, D.J., McCary, J.D., and Raffa, R.B. A response surface analysis of synergism between morphine and clonidine. *J. Pharmacol. Exp. Ther.* 289:8–13, 1999.

Tallarida, R.J., Stone, D.J., and Raffa, R.B. Efficient designs for studying synergistic drug combinations. *Life Sci.* 61:PL417–425, 1997.

Wilcox, G.L., Carlsson, K.H., Jochim, A., and Jurna, I. Mutual potentiation of antinociceptive effects of morphine and clonidine on motor and sensory responses in rat spinal cord. *Brain Res.* 405:84–93, 1987.

Nonlinear Regression Analysis

Thus far we have illustrated the use of linear regression as a way of fitting dose-effect data. When the effect is plotted against the logarithm of the dose over some mid-range of doses, a somewhat linear trend often results. In this limited dose range, the points are often well approximated by a straight line fit; thus, if there are sufficient points in this linear region, the use of linear regression is often adequate to get D_{50} values and their standard errors. However, the complete log dose-effect curve, that is, the curve over an extensive range of log dose values, is frequently sigmoidal (S-shaped) and, thus, nonlinear.

In binary outcomes (quantal data) the sigmoidal curve is analyzed by transforming to probits (or logits) as we saw in Chapter 6. This transformation often produces an acceptable linear fit of the data. For graded (continuous) dose-effect data, probit analysis is not employed as an analytical procedure (even though it often straightens the sigmoid curve). Graded data will often fit a hyperbolic curve (also nonlinear) when the effect is plotted against the dose over the entire dose range. This was illustrated in Chapter 2 where we used the hyperbolic function, $E = E_{max}D/(D + C)$, to describe the graded dose-effect relation and in Chapter 10 where we saw its application to the drugs clonidine and morphine.

The double reciprocal plot, $1/E$ against $1/D$, has been frequently used when data are presumed to be hyperbolic, a use that is common in the analysis of enzyme substrate kinetics. The basis for this is easily seen by rearranging the hyperbola to give $1/E = 1/E_{max} + (C/E_{max})\, 1/D$. This is theoretically linear in the reciprocated variables, $1/E$ and $1/D$, with slope $= C/E_{max}$ and intercept $= 1/E_{max}$. But reciprocated variables are not suitable for linear regression analysis (other than as first approximations), and, thus, the parameter estimates obtained this way are questionable; also, there is no acceptable way to get their variances.

With the availability of personal computers in recent years, a number of software packages have appeared that allow the user to select a nonlinear modeling equation that contains the parameters needed, such as E_{max} and D_{50}. (*The companion software package to this book contains such a program*; *see page 204*.) In this procedure, the user makes an *initial estimate* of the needed parameters, and the program calculates the best-fitting value of the parameters while also providing estimates of their standard errors. The mathematical basis of the technique is in Taylor series. An outline of the idea and a demonstration are given below. But first we describe the functional forms that are most often employed in describing dose-effect data. Also described are the usual transformations.

Simple hyperbolic

This form is given by $E = E_{max} D/(D + C)$ and the Taylor series approach allows an estimate of both E_{max} and C ($= D_{50}$) from the (D, E) data points. Usually five or more points are needed for data that show a smooth trend. Very often the fit is acceptable and the E_{max} and C values are also acceptable based on the standard error estimates that are obtained. When the standard errors appear to be too large, it may be necessary to first transform the data to a form suitable to the *Hill equation*.

11.1   Hill equation

The Hill equation is obtained as a transformation of the hyperbolic form, $E = E_{max}D/(D + C)$ and has found much use in the analysis of the oxygen saturation of hemoglobin, where an exponent p is put on D and C, and also in the analysis of radioligand binding sites. Our use here is for curve fitting. When $p = 1$ the Hill equation is a simple transformation of the hyperbolic relation expressed in logarithmic form:

$$\log\left(\frac{E}{E_{max} - E}\right) = \log D - \log C \qquad (11.1)$$

Instead of plotting E against D, this form requires plotting the logarithm of $E/(E_{max} - E)$ against the logarithm of D. When this plot is made, the graph is a straight line with unit slope and vertical intercept $= -\log C$. When applied to actual data, the points are fitted to a straight line. This is a useful plot because getting a slope other than one provides some indication of the adequacy of the hyperbolic model. If the slope differs significantly from one, then the hyperbolic model will not give a good fit to the data. In such cases, the Hill plot *slope*, denoted p, suggests a different (better-fitting) equation such as

$$E = \frac{E_{max}D^p}{D^p + C^p}.$$ (11.2)

Of course, the transformation of the data that led to the Hill plot requires that E_{max} is known, yet that is one of the values to be estimated from the data. When the data have been appropriately normalized to $E_{max} = 100\%$, then that value is used as E_{max} in this plot. In other cases a reasonable estimate of E_{max} must be made so that the plot can be generated and the slope estimated. A series of successive approximations may be necessary. That is, one makes a guess at E_{max} so that the data are transformed to quantities $\log (E/(E_{max} - E))$ for the y-axis. A plot of these against $\log D$ would then be described by

$$\log\left(\frac{E}{E_{max} - E}\right) = p\log D - p\log C.$$ (11.3)

Equation 11.3 is seen to be a line with slope p in the transformed variables. Thus, one uses the Hill plot to get the slope which is then used as the value of p in Equation 11.2. With p inserted into Equation 11.2 one can proceed to fit the data to this equation. If the fit is acceptable, then both E_{max} and C are calculated. If the fit still seems unacceptable, then the value of p can be adjusted upward or downward. An application of that procedure is given in the following example (Table 11.1).

Example. Data from Table 2.1 were transformed, as shown in Table 11.1, in order to construct the Hill plot of Figure 11.1. For this purpose E_{max} was taken to be 20. Regression analysis gave slope = 1.44 ± 0.078; accordingly, p was taken = 1.4 and E_{max} = 20 in Equation 11.2. This analysis produced the plot shown in Figure 11.2. This fitted curve gave $D_{50} = 16.3 \pm 0.38 \times 10^{-7}$ M.

11.2 Theory

The basis of nonlinear curve fitting is as follows. A function E of concentration z contains, say, two parameters (E_{max} and D_{50}), denoted

Table 11.1. Methoxamine Data of Table 2.1 Transformed for Hill Plot*

D	E	(Em − E)	E/(Em − E)	log D	log[E/(Em − E)]
1.40	0.196	19.8	0.00990	0.146	−2.00
2.30	0.588	19.4	0.0303	0.362	−1.52
4.10	1.96	18.0	0.109	0.613	−0.964
5.70	3.33	16.7	0.200	0.756	−0.699
8.00	5.48	14.5	0.377	0.903	−0.423
11.0	7.84	12.2	0.645	1.04	−0.191
15.0	9.60	10.4	0.923	1.18	−0.0348
23.0	12.5	7.50	1.67	1.36	0.222
39.0	15.3	4.70	3.26	1.59	0.513
53.0	16.8	3.20	5.25	1.72	0.720
80.0	18.0	2.00	9.00	1.90	0.954
170	19.2	0.800	24.0	2.23	1.38
420	19.4	0.600	32.3	2.62	1.51

* Concentration, M × 10^7 ; E in millinewtons. Doses values ×10^{-7} (values rounded).

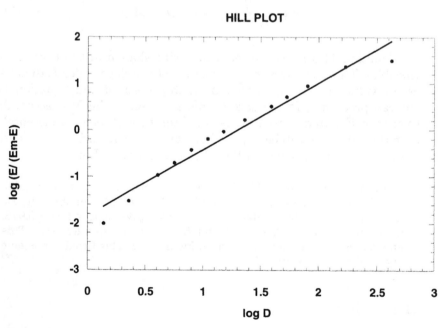

Figure 11.1. Hill plot for methoxamine-induced contraction in aortic strips (see Table 11.1).

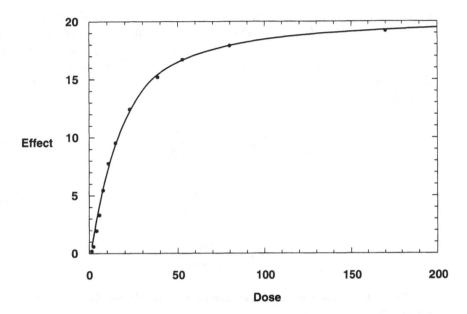

Figure 11.2. Dose-effect data from Table 11.1 are fitted to Equation 11.2 for $p = 1.4$.

here by α and β, that is, $E = f(z, \alpha, \beta)$. We seek here a representation in which α and β are estimated by a and b. These estimates are initially a_0 and b_0. A Taylor series representation is made about these initial estimates a_0 and b_0:

$$E \approx f(a_0, b_0, z) + (\partial f / \partial \alpha)(\alpha - a_0) + (\partial f / \partial \beta)(\beta - b_0) \qquad (11.4)$$

$$E - f(a_0, b_0, z) \approx (\partial f / \partial \alpha)(\alpha - a_0) + (\partial f / \partial \beta)(\beta - b_0). \qquad (11.5)$$

For this choice of a_0 for α and b_0 for β, each dose value z_i gives the left-hand side of Equation 11.5, $E_i - f(a_0, b_0, z_i)$, denoted here by Y_{res}. Further, the partial derivative $\partial f / \partial \alpha$ uses the a_0 an b_0 values and also has a value for each z_i value, denoted here by $X1_i$. Similarly, the partial derivative $\partial f / \partial \beta$ has a value at this z_i which we denote by $X2_i$. Thus, we get a set of values of a dependent variable Y_{res} that is linearly related to the independent variables $X1$ and $X2$. A multiple linear regression (see Chapter 12) yields the two regression coefficients $\alpha - a_0$ and $\beta - b_0$.

The following applies this mathematical algorithm for estimating parameters α and β in a hyperbolic model, $Y = \alpha x/(x + \beta)$ for the dose-response data set, (x_i, y_i). (Note that the dose is now denoted by x.) Thus, $E_{max} = \alpha$ and $D_{50} = \beta$. The partial derivatives are $\partial f / \partial \alpha = x/(x + \beta)$ and $\partial f / \partial \beta = -\alpha x/(x + \beta)^2$. There are N data points. Original estimates of parameters are denoted a_0 and b_0. The data are transformed into three different sets, denoted by Y_{res}, X_1, and X_2, defined as follows:

$$Y_{res} = y_i - \frac{a_0 x_i}{x_i + b_0} \tag{11.6}$$

$$X_1 = \frac{x_i}{x_i + b_0} \tag{11.7}$$

$$X_2 = \frac{-a_0 x_i}{(x_i + b_0)^2}. \tag{11.8}$$

Thus, the original data set gives rise to three data columns of length N:

Y_{res}	X_1	X_2
...	...	...
...	...	...

The values of Y_{res}, X_1, and X_2, in the above array are entered into a standard linear multiple regression program modeled as

$$Y_{res} = cX_1 + d\,X_2. \tag{11.9}$$

Multiple linear regression is a standard procedure that is contained in certain software packages,* and details applicable to our application are given in Chapter 12. The coefficients c and d are determined (with standard errors) from these programs, and these allow improved estimates of parameters a and b by taking a new set of estimates:

$$a_1 = c + a_0$$

and

$$b_1 = d + b_0.$$

*See p. 204.

The new set of estimates, a_1 and b_1 are entered into Equations 11.6 to 11.8 (in place of a_0 and b_0) and the linear regression program to yield a_2 and b_2 (with std. errors). A stopping criterion is applied, e.g., if the difference between two iterates is < 0.01. This last set is retained and the last set's standard errors are retained as the standard errors of the final estimate.

11.3 Sigmoid plot

Many dose-effect curves take on a sigmoid (S) shape when the effect is plotted against the logarithm of the dose. The basis of this shape is best understood in relation to the "logistic curve" which was mentioned in Chapter 6. Some additional discussion is given here.

The logistic curve arises in certain biological problems, such as the growth of populations, and is often a topic in the study of differential equations. Discussions of these applications may be found in Rainville and Bedient (1989) and Weisstein (1999). For our purposes, the form of the logistic function is given by

$$y = \frac{A}{1 + B.10^{-x}} \tag{11.10}$$

where A and B are constants. Note that as x increases, y approaches A, whereas as x decreases (approaches negative infinity), y approaches zero. In the application at hand, A is the maximum effect of the drug, B is the D_{50}, $x = \log D$, and $y =$ effect. To see this more clearly, we start with the hyperbolic form, $y = AD/(D + B)$, and the identity, $D = 10^{\log D} = 10^x$; then, effect $y = ((A.10^x)/(10^x + B)) = (A/(1 + B.10^{-x}))$. Therefore a plot of y against x is a plot of effect against $\log D$. When a slope factor p is needed, the equation becomes $y = ((A.10^{px})/(10^{px} + B^p))$. This form was applied to the data $(\log D, E) = (x, y)$, of Table 11.1 in which we took $p = 1.4$ and $A = 20$. The resulting graph is shown, with the data points, in Figure 11.3. The curve-fitting procedure gave $B = 16.28$ which is the D_{50} for these data (see example Section 11.1).

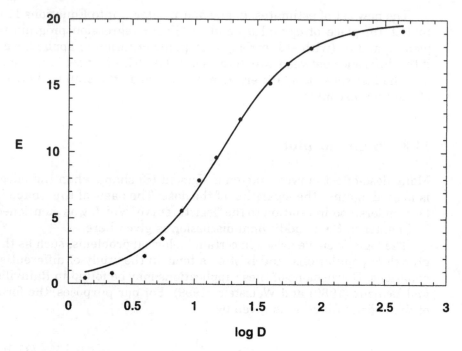

Figure 11.3. Methoxamine data from Table 11.1, graphed as E against $\log D$, and the smooth sigmoid curve given $y = ((A.10^{px})/(10^{px} + B^p))$ with $p = 1.4$.

CHAPTER 11

References

Rainville, E.D. and Bedient, P.E. *Elementary Differential Equations,* 7th ed. Macmillan, New York, 1989.

Weisstein, E.W. *CRC Concise Encyclopedia of Mathematics.* Chapman & Hall/CRC, Boca Raton, 1999.

Statistical Concepts
and Tests of Hypotheses

12.1 Hypothesis testing with the *t*-test: two groups

The *t*-test was discussed previously in connection with dose-effect data and distinguishing between the $\log D_{50}$ values from two curves or the $\log ED50$ values from two curves (see Chapter 4). This test is also very widely used for comparing the group means of two samples, $\{x_1, x_2, ..., x_{n1}\}$ containing n_1 elements and $\{y_1, y_2, ..., y_{n2}\}$ containing n_2 elements. True standard deviations of each population are often unknown and are estimated from the sample standard deviations, s_x and s_y, calculated from the respective variances (square of *s* values). The formulas for the sample means and variances are familiar to most readers:

$$\bar{x} = \frac{\sum x_i}{n_1} \quad \text{and} \quad \bar{y} = \frac{\sum y_i}{n_2} \tag{12.1}$$

$$s_x^2 = \frac{\sum (x_i - \bar{x})^2}{n_1 - 1} \quad \text{and} \quad s_y^2 = \frac{\sum (y_i - \bar{y})^2}{n_2 - 1}. \tag{12.2}$$

An alternate equation for calculating a variance (say s_x^2) is

$$s_x^2 = \frac{\sum r_i^2 - n_i \bar{x}^2}{n_1 - 1}. \tag{12.3}$$

A similar formula, of course, applies to s_y^2.

In applying the *t*-test these variances are used to get a pooled estimate, s^2, computed from

$$s^2 = \frac{(n_1 - 1)^2 s_x^2 + (n_2 - 1)^2 s_y^2}{n_1 + n_2 - 2}. \tag{12.4}$$

The quantity calculated as

$$t = \frac{\bar{x} - \bar{y}}{s \sqrt{\dfrac{1}{n_1} + \dfrac{1}{n_2}}} \tag{12.5}$$

follows the t-distribution with $n_1 + n_2 - 2$ degrees of freedom if the two population means are equal. This equality is the null hypothesis and a rejection of this hypothesis tells us, in simpler language, that the two means differ significantly. Accordingly the quantity calculated from Equation 12.5 must exceed in magnitude the value in Table A.6. The following example illustrates this application.

Example. Isometric force in isolated aortic strips of the rabbit was measured in response to a fixed dose of norepinephrine. In one set of experiments, the passive tension (preload) was set low, whereas in the other it was set at a higher value. Force was in millinewtons and was converted to grams for listing below. The lower preload group is denoted by X and the higher by Y in Table 12.1 which also shows pertinent statistics.

Table 12.1. Force Development in Isolated Aortic Strips*

Sets	X	Y
	1.9	2.4
	2.3	3.1
	2.6	3.5
	2.7	4.0
	2.8	3.9
	2.2	4.1
		4.4
		4.8
Sum	14.5	30.2
Number (n)	6	8
Mean	2.4167	3.775
Std Deviation	0.3430	0.7592
Variance	0.1177	0.5764
Std Error	0.1400	0.2684

* Unpublished data, MacNab and Tallarida.

The pooled variance is

$$s^2 = \frac{(6-1)(0.1177) + (8-1)(0.5764)}{12}$$

$$= 0.3853.$$

Thus, $s = 0.6207$ and this value is used in the calculation of t from Equation 12.5:

$$t = \frac{2.4167 - 3.775}{0.6207\sqrt{\frac{1}{6} + \frac{1}{8}}} = -4.052.$$

From Table A.6, for 12 degrees of freedom (99% level), the critical $t = 3.055$. Since the calculated t has a *magnitude* greater than 3.055 we may conclude that the difference is significant; i.e., we reject with appreciable confidence the hypothesis that the two populations are the same. (See also, Equations 4.7 and 4.8.)

The t-test is based on the assumption that the *data are normal* (see Figure 6.2 and discussion in Chapter 6). When the number of objects in each group is large, say > 30, we are less concerned about this assumption because of a certain theoretical result (the central limit theorem) which ensures that the sample means are approximately normal regardless of the underlying distribution. But even for small samples, it has been shown that, unless the departure from normality is extreme, or the number of objects is very small, this distribution is insensitive to even moderate departures from normality. In other words, the t-test is a robust test of significance, and this property accounts for its widespread use. Nevertheless there are situations in which the assumptions of the t-test may not apply. Such situations sometimes occur in certain behavioral tests in animals. This concern has prompted the development of distribution-free tests (nonparametric tests) for examining the differences in two groups. One such test that is quite popular (Mann-Whitney) is discussed subsequently. Before this, we discuss the paired t-test.

12.2 t-test: paired data

It is often possible to pair the values obtained in two different situations. For example, data might consist of measurements on the same subject under two different conditions. In such cases it is the difference in the values that is important. This situation frequently occurs in drug testing; for example, when each animal provides a value (say, heart rate) before drug administration and after drug administration. An example is indicated in the data of Table 12.2. The null hypothesis is that the mean difference is zero. The set of n differences (d's) are used to get the mean $\bar{d}$ and the standard deviation s_d from which t is calculated from the following equations:

$$\bar{d} = \frac{\sum d_i}{n} \tag{12.6}$$

$$s_d = \sqrt{\frac{\sum (d_i - \bar{d})^2}{n-1}} \tag{12.7}$$

$$t = \frac{\bar{d}}{s_d / \sqrt{n}} \tag{12.8}$$

The degrees of freedom $= n - 1$ in this application of the t-test and this number is needed in using Table A.6. If the calculated t exceeds the tabular value then the difference is significant. For the data in the following example (Table 12.2) the mean difference is 6.125 and is seen to be significant ($p < 0.05$).

Table 12.2. Heart Rates Before and After Drug Administration

	Before Treatment	After Treatment	Difference
	88	94	6
	93	108	15
	87	89	2
	105	119	14
	91	98	7
	80	84	4
	101	100	−1
	85	87	2
Mean	6.125		
Std Deviation	5.743		
Variance	32.98		
Std Error	2.030	$t = 3.017$	$t_{0.05} = 2.365$

Example. The data in Table 12.2, from a student animal laboratory exercise, give the heart rates in the same animal before and after a small dose of isoproterenol, a *beta* adrenoceptor stimulating drug.

12.3 Confidence interval

Besides its use in comparing two groups, the t–distribution has an important use in calculating confidence limits of the mean. When n values are obtained from a normal variate with mean μ and variance σ^2, a 95% confidence interval is calculated from the sample mean $\bar{x}$ as $\bar{x} \pm 1.96\sigma/\sqrt{n}$. Usually we do not know the variance σ^2, but have only the sample standard deviation s_x. In this case it is necessary to replace the number 1.96 (from the standard normal curve) by a value of the t-distribution (for $n - 1$ degrees of freedom). Thus, the population mean lies between $\bar{x} \pm ts_x/\sqrt{n}$. This is called a *confidence interval*. For the set of differences in Table 12.2, the mean difference = 6.125 and $s_x/\sqrt{n}$ = 2.030; hence, using the t-value 2.365 (for 95% and *d.f.* = 7) from appendix Table A.6, we calculate the confidence interval to be 6.125 ± 4.801.

12.4 Mann-Whitney test

The Mann-Whitney test is a nonparametric test to compare two populations. As in the t-test, the entries from groups 1 and 2 will generally have unequal numbers, denoted by n_1 and n_2. Sample data are shown in Table 12.3. We wish to determine if the means of the two groups are different.

Table 12.3. Data for Mann-Whitney Test

Group #1	Group #2
1	2
8	12
9	14
12	16
	23
$(n_1 = 4)$	$(n_2 = 5)^*$

* In cases of unequal sample size, n_2 is taken to be the larger.

The elements from both sets are arranged in ascending order and that order has a rank number (R) listed below; thus

Number	**1**	**2**	**8**	**9**	**12**	12	14	16	23
Rank	(1)	(2)	(3)	(4)	(5.5)	(5.5)	(7)	(8)	(9)

Note that the number 12 occurs in positions 5 and 6; rather than rank these differently, we give each of them the average rank, 5.5. Note also that we have distinguished the elements by writing those from set #1 with bold type. This allows us to easily identify the set from which each element came and its rank number. The *ranks* of set #1 elements are summed and those from set #2 are summed to give quantities, R_1 and R_2, respectively:

$$R_1 = 1 + 3 + 4 + 5.5 = 13.5$$

$$R_2 = 2 + 5.5 + 7 + 8 + 9 = 31.5$$

From these rank sums we calculate U_1 and U_2 from the following:

$$U_1 = n_1 n_2 + \frac{n_1(n_1 + 1)}{2} - R_1 \qquad (12.9)$$

$$U_2 = n_1 n_2 + \frac{n_2(n_2 + 1)}{2} - R_2 \qquad (12.10)$$

In this example, $n_2 = 5$ and $n_1 = 4$. From Equations 12.9 and 12.10, $U_1 = 16.5$ and $U_2 = 3.5$.

The statistic U is taken to be the smaller of U_1 and U_2 and its value, along with the values of n_1 and n_2 allow the use of tables from which the significance of the difference is judged. There are two sets of tables in the appendix (A11a and A11b) and the choice depends on the set sizes.

Case 1

If neither n_1 nor n_2 is larger than 8, we use Table A.11a which uses n_1, n_2 and the calculated U to give a probability. Significance is indicated by a small p, e.g., $p < 0.05$ is required to show a difference.

Case 2

If n_2 is greater than 8, then Table A.11b is used. In this table, the numbers n_1 and n_2 are used for the significance level (e.g., $p < 0.05$) and the table values give the critical value of U. If the calculated U is less than or equal to the tabular U, the difference is significant.

In our example (Table 12.3) $U = 3.5$ and, because n_2 is not larger than 8, we use Table A.11a with this value of U and $n_1 = 4$, $n_2 = 5$. It is seen that the p value is a number between 0.056 and 0.095. Since this number is not less than 0.05 (usual criterion for significance) we cannot conclude that there is a significant difference.

We now illustrate using a group that has more than eight elements, along with a group containing four elements. We also have selected the values to demonstrate the smallness of U in cases of very high significance. Thus, let one set be {4, 5, 6, 8} and the other {7, 9, 11, 12, 16, 18, 20, 21, 22}. The rank sums are $R_1 = 11$ and $R_2 = 80$ and, from Equations 12.9 and 12.10, $U_1 = 35$ and $U_2 = 1$; thus $U = 1$. From table A-11b, the critical value of $U(p < 0.05)$ is 4. Because the calculated U is less than 4, the difference is significant. In fact, the difference is seen to be significant (from the table value) for $p = 0.02$.

12.5   Analysis of variance

When the means of two samples are to be compared, we use the t-test (or the Mann-Whitney test). When there are three or more sets of data (for example, k sets), the comparison of means is first accomplished with the analysis of variance (ANOVA) which uses the F-distribution. It may seem correct to use individual t-tests on each pair of means; this usage, however, can lead to wrong conclusions and is not recommended. Analysis of variance, described here, is the recommended procedure.

In our description we denote the number of elements in the k sets by n_1, n_2, ..., n_k . The data array is depicted in Table 12.4. The k sets are arranged in columns and the elements (the B's) have a double subscript (*row, column*) as shown in Table 12.4. The individual sample means, $\bar{B}_1, \bar{B}_2, ..., \bar{B}_k$, for the k sets are computed, as is the *grand mean* $\bar{B}$. The grand mean is used to calculate quantities denoted SS, SST, and SSE. First, every element in the entire array is reduced by the grand mean and each reduced quantity is squared and summed to form the quantity SS:

Table 12.4. Data Array for Use in Analysis of Variance

Sample 1	Sample 2	. . .	Sample k
$B_{1,1}$	$B_{1,2}$		$B_{1,k}$
$B_{2,1}$	$B_{2,2}$		$B_{2,k}$
.	.		.
.	.		.
.	.		.
$B_{n1,1}$			
			$B_{nk,k}$
	.		
	$B_{n2,2}$		
$\bar{B}_1$	$\bar{B}_2$		$\bar{B}_k$ *(means)*

$$\bar{B} = \frac{\sum \bar{B}_i}{k} \quad \textit{(grand mean)}$$

$$SS = (B_{1,1} - \bar{B})^2 + (B_{2,1} - \bar{B})^2 + ...(B_{nk,k} - \bar{B})^2. \qquad (12.11)$$

Also needed are quantities SST and SSE defined as follows:

$$SST = n_1(\bar{B}_1 - \bar{B})^2 + n_2(\bar{B}_2 - \bar{B})^2 + ... + n_k(\bar{B}_k - \bar{B})^2 \qquad (12.12)$$

$$SSE = \sum(B_{i1} - \bar{B}_1)^2 + \sum(B_{i2} - \bar{B}_2)^2 + ... + \sum(B_{ik} - \bar{B}_k)^2. \qquad (12.13)$$

SSE is formed by summing the squares of each element in the column reduced by the column mean; therefore, it is called the *within sample sum of squares*. SST involves the sum of squares of column means, reduced by the grand mean; it is called the *between means sum of squares*. It measures the dispersion of the sample means about the grand mean. These quantities are related by

$$SS = SST + SSE. \qquad (12.14)$$

These provide two estimates of the population variance, denoted s_p^2 and s_t^2 :

$$s_p^2 = \frac{SSE}{n_1 + n_2 + \ldots + n_k - k} \qquad (12.15)$$

and

$$s_t^2 = \frac{SST}{k-1}. \qquad (12.16)$$

The ratio of these follows the F-distribution,

$$F = \frac{s_t^2}{s_p^2} \qquad (12.17)$$

with degrees of freedom $k - 1$ (across) and $n_1 + n_2 + \ldots + n_k - k$ (down). Table A.9 gives the values of F. If the calculated F exceeds the tabular value, then at least one pair of the group means differ significantly. (In the special case of $k = 2$, that is, when two groups are being compared, it may be shown that the value of F is the square of t used in Student's t-test.) The results of this analysis are usually arranged in a table such as Table 12.5. A worked example is given in the next section. While the calculation of F may show that one or more differences exists among the means, it does not identify the group or groups responsible. To find out which pair (or pairs) differ significantly, we can use a test known as Newman-Keuls test.

Table 12.5. Analysis of Variance for Unequal Sample Sizes

Source	Sum of squares	D.F.*	Mean square	F
Total	SS	v_1		
Between	SST	v_2	$s_t^2 = \dfrac{SST}{v_2}$	$\dfrac{s_t^2}{s_p^2} = F$
Within	SSE	v_3	$s_p^2 = \dfrac{SSE}{v_3}$	

* $v_1 = \left(\sum n_i\right) - 1$; $v_2 = k - 1$; $v_3 = \left(\sum n_i\right) - k$

12.6   Newman-Keuls test

When the F-test indicates a significant difference the Newman-Keuls Test examines the k sample means. These are arranged in order of *increasing magnitude*

$$\bar{B}_1, \bar{B}_2, ..., \bar{B}_k .$$

Note that this notation now denotes increasing magnitude and is not the same as the group numbers 1, 2, ..., k in the preceding discussion of analysis of variance. For the largest and the smallest means, we calculate the quantity q given by

$$q = \frac{\bar{B}_k - \bar{B}_1}{SE} \tag{12.18}$$

where

$$SE = \left[\frac{(s_p)^2}{2} \left(\frac{1}{n_k} + \frac{1}{n_1} \right) \right]^{1/2} . \tag{12.19}$$

The number q calculated from these equations is associated with an integer w that equals the number of means in the range of this pair; in this case, $w = k$. The next calculation considers the largest against the "second smallest," i.e., $\bar{B}_k$ and $\bar{B}_2$ are used to form SE and q, using numbers n_k and n_2. Now the associated number $w = k$-1, since this is the number of means in the range 2 to k. Subsequent calculations are for the remaining pairs: largest against third smallest, etc., then second largest against smallest, etc., thereby considering all combinations of two means.

For any pair of means, appendix Table A.10 is used to get the critical value of q to which the calculated q is compared. The table value depends on degrees of freedom, given by $d.f. = (n_1 + n_2 + ... + n_k - k)$, and the value of w that is appropriate for the pair under consideration. The tables are given for confidence levels 95% and 99%. *If the calculated q for any pair $\geq$ tabular value, then the difference between those means is significant.* We provide an example below, with made-up numbers, in order to simplify the illustration.

Table 12.6. Differences Among Means

	I	II	III	IV
	3	16	21	4
	6	8	25	6
	8	3	20	7
	5	9		6
		14		
mean	5.5	10	22	5.75

grand mean = 10.8125

$SS = 731.9375$	$s_p^2 = 11.4792$	
$SSE = 137.75$	$s_t^2 = 198.0625$	$F_{3, 12} = 5.95$ (99%)
$SST = 594.1875$	$F = 17.254$	$F_{3, 12} = 3.49$ (95%)

Example. Four groups have the values given in Table 12.6. It is desired to test for differences among the means and to determine which pairs of means, if any, are significantly different. It is seen that the calculated F value exceeds the tabular value (99%); thus the means differ. To determine which pairs are significantly different we apply the Newman-Keuls test. To do this we arrange the four means in ascending order:

5.5	5.75	10	22
(4)	(4)	(5)	(3)

The number of objects (n_i) in each group is shown below each mean. Table 12.7 lists the six pairs and the calculated values of SE and q, as well as the value of w that are needed for use of Table A.10. It is noted that $d.f.$ = 12 in this application. Among the pairs of means listed, the first three differ significantly (in each case, $p < 0.01$) and these are indicated by **; the other three did not reach significance even at the 0.05 level.

Table 12.7. Newman-Keuls Analysis

pair	SE	w	q
22/5.5	1.830	4	9.016**
22/5.75	1.830	3	8.880**
22/10	1.749	2	6.861**
10/5.5	1.607	3	2.800
10/5.75	1.607	2	2.645
5.75/5.5	1.694	2	0.148

12.7   Chi square

If n events occur with observed frequencies $o_1, o_2, ..., o_n$ and their corresponding expected frequencies are $e_1, e_2, ..., e_n$, the *chi square* statistic, denoted χ^2, is given by

$$\chi^2 = \sum_1^n \frac{(o_i - e_i)^2}{e_i}. \tag{12.20}$$

The calculation of χ^2 provides a number that indicates the agreement between the observed and the expected frequencies. A small value of this statistic means good agreement between the observed and expected frequencies of the n events. The distribution of chi square is associated with a constant, the degrees of freedom (*d.f.*). For the n events considered above *d.f.* $= n - 1$. The appendix Table A.7 gives the value of this statistic for different degrees of freedom at both the 95% and the 99% significance levels.

The analysis of dose-effect data often leads to situations in which a characteristic is classified into classes represented in rows (R) and a second characteristic is also classified into classes expressed in columns (C). A row-column entry constitutes a cell, and each cell contains a number. For example, three different species of an animal may respond or not respond to a drug (Table 12.8). This is an example of a *contingency table*. The species, denoted I, II, and III, showed responses and non-responses as shown, and it is desired to determine whether the relative numbers of responders is the same across the three strains.

In other words, is the response independent of the strain? The entries in the table constitute the observed numbers; the expected numbers are computed under the assumption that there is no difference. For example, in group I, while the observed number of responders is 12, the expected number of responders, if all strains were equal, is 32/153 times the number (52) in group I. Thus, 32 × 52/153 = 10.9. Then in this group, the expected number of nonresponders = 52 ×

Table 12.8. Contingency Table

	I	II	III	Totals
Response	12	14	6	32
No response	40	40	41	121
	52	54	47	**153**

121/153 = 41.1. (Of course, the sum of responders and nonresponders is the group total 52). The expected number for each cell is (*row-total*) × (*column-total*)/*total*. Proceeding in this way, we get for each cell observed and expected pairs, (o_i, e_i), as follows: (12, 10.9), (14, 11.3), (6, 9.8), (40, 41.1), (40, 42.7), (41, 37.2). A significant difference among the strains is indicated by a large value of χ^2 calculated from Equation 12.20, i.e., a value that is greater than the critical value in Table A.7. In this kind of application of chi square (contingency table) the degrees of freedom = $(R - 1) \times (C - 1)$. Thus, in this example, *d.f.* = 2. From Equation 12.20, $\chi^2 = 2.84$. This calculated value is compared with the value in Table A.7 for 2 degrees of freedom. The table value (for 95% confidence) is 5.99. Because the calculated value does not exceed the tabular value, we cannot conclude that there is a significant difference among the three strains.

Adjusted chi square

In a 2 × 2 contingency table, *d.f.* = 1. In this situation an adjustment, called the "Yate's correction," is needed and it computes chi square according to

$$\chi^2 = \sum \frac{(|o_i - e_i| - 1/2)^2}{e_i}.$$ (12.21)

Comparing two proportions

The form of the chi square given by Equation 12.21 is applicable to comparisons of two proportions and is illustrated in the following example.

> **Example.** Two drugs are tested for a response (all or none) in laboratory animals. Drug #1 produces a response in 12 of 15 animals (80%), whereas drug 2 is found to be effective in only 6 of 10 animals (60%) tested. The test results may be expressed in the 2×2 contingency table shown in Table 12.9.
>
> Since this is a 2×2 contingency table there is one degree of freedom. The calculated $\chi^2 = 0.405$ from Equation 12.21, and it does not exceed the tabular value 3.84 of Table A.7 (for 95% level). Thus, the difference is not significant. This example points out the difficulty of drawing conclu-

Table 12.9. Contingency Table for Testing Two Proportions

	I	II	Totals
Response	12	6	18
No response	3	4	7
	15	10	**25**

sions based on single dose experimentation. Many more animals would have to be tested (discussed subsequently) even to show a difference as large as the 20% suggested in this example. This finding emphasizes the need for dose-effect analysis, i.e., the use of several doses, and the regression and other models discussed in earlier chapters.

12.8   Confidence limits of a proportion

When N subjects are treated with a drug and L of them respond, we estimate the proportion of responders, $p = L/N$, as indicative of the population. But the estimated proportion p has a variance and, therefore, the estimate requires confidence limits. When N is large, say greater than 30, confidence limits are calculated from

$$p \pm Z\sqrt{p(1-p)/N} \tag{12.22}$$

where Z is taken from the standard normal curve as 1.96 (95% limits) or 2.58 (99% limits). For smaller values of N, the confidence limits are values computed from

$$\frac{N}{N+Z_2}\{p - 1/(2N) + Z^2/(2N) - Z\sqrt{R_1}\} \tag{12.23}$$

and

$$\frac{N}{N+Z_2}\{p + 1/(2N) + Z^2/(2N) + Z\sqrt{R_2}\}. \tag{12.24}$$

In these formulas R_1 and R_2 are given by

$$R_1 = [p + 1/(2N)][1 - p - 1/(2N)] / N + Z^2/(4N^2) \tag{12.25}$$

$$R_2 = [p - 1/(2N)][(1 - p + 1/(2N)] / N + Z^2/(4N^2). \tag{12.26}$$

In using these formulas it is recommended that $Np > 5$ and $N(1-p) > 5$.

> **Example.** In a drug trial that tested 20 subjects it was observed that 8 showed a favorable response; thus p = 0.4. Substitution of these values in the above equations, using $Z = 1.96$ (for 95% confidence limits), gives limits of 0.196 to 0.632. If 40 subjects were tested and gave the same proportion (16 responders) the calculation shows that the confidence limits narrow to 0.251 to 0.564. This example again points out the statistical challenge when dealing with a single dose.

12.9   Confidence limits for a ratio

It is often necessary in pharmacological investigations to consider the ratio of two variables. For example, the relative potency of two drugs is the ratio of their D_{50} values or *ED50* values. In considering a ratio, it is clear that both the numerator and the denominator are estimated quantities, and, thus, the ratio of these has confidence limits. In other words, the parameters α and β give a ratio $\mu = \alpha/\beta$ that is estimated by measured quantities a and b, so the ratio is estimated as a/b. We wish to determine the limits within which μ lies. This question was addressed by Cochran (1938) and by Finney (1964), but the definitive result is due to Fieller (1944), whose result is given here in an expression for the limits. Provided that the *numerator and denominator are independent* the confidence limits are given by

$$\frac{a}{b} + \frac{g}{(1-g)}\left(\frac{a}{b}\right) \pm \frac{t}{b(1-g)}\sqrt{V(a) + \frac{a^2}{b^2}V(b) - gV(a)} \qquad (12.27)$$

where

$$g = \frac{t^2 V(b)}{b^2}. \qquad (12.28)$$

If the individual means come from n_1 and n_2 values, respectively, and if the individual variances can be pooled, then t has d.f. $= n_1 + n_2 - 2$. If the values of the numerator and denominator are D_{50} or *ED50* values from regression analysis, say parallel line estimates (Chapter 3), then d.f. $= n_1 + n_2 - 3$. If these are the results of probit analysis (Chapter 6) the value of t depends on the value of g.

If g is small, say, less than 0.1, t has the value from the normal distribution (1.96 for 95% confidence limits); when g cannot be neglected, then t is a value from the *Student* distribution (Table A.6).

Note that when g can be neglected, the second term of Equation 12.27 is

$$\pm t \sqrt{\frac{V(a)}{a^2} + \frac{a^2}{b^4}V(b)} = \pm t\frac{a}{b}\sqrt{\frac{V(a)}{b^2} + \frac{V(b)}{b^2}}.$$

Accordingly, the coefficient of t "looks like" a standard error, and this quantity is sometimes used as an approximation for the standard error of a quotient when the numerator and denominator are independent (have zero covariance):

$$SE\left(\frac{a}{b}\right) \approx \frac{a}{b}\sqrt{\frac{V(a)}{a^2} + \frac{V(b)}{b^2}}. \tag{12.29}$$

Example. If $a = 20$ with standard deviation 4 and $b = 6$ with standard deviation 3, the variances $V(a) = 16$ and $V(b) = 9$, inserted into the above equation, lead to $SE(a/b) = 1.79$.

12.10 Multiple regression (equations)

In our discussion on nonlinear curve-fitting (Chapter 11) we saw the need for iterative use of 2–parameter linear regression given by

$$Y = b_1 X_1 + b_2 X_2$$

At every step of the iterative process, a set of X_1, X_2, and corresponding Y values (there denoted by Y_{res}) were calculated, and, at that step, we wish to calculate the coefficients b_1 and b_2. The procedure for doing this is a special case of the general multiple regression algorithm based on $Y = b_0 + b_1 X_1 + b_2 X_2 + \ldots + b_n X_n$, that estimates all the coefficients. In our application (2–parameter nonlinear analysis) there is no b_0 term and $n = 2$. The data array is that shown in Table 12.10.

Our model equation is

$$\hat{Y} = b_1 X_1 + b_2 X_2. \tag{12.30}$$

Table 12.10. Data Array for a Step in Nonlinear Curve Fitting Procedure

Data	Y	X_1	X_2
	...	...	...
	...	...	...
(n sets)	at each cycle of the procedure		

The least squares procedure leads to "normal equations" whose solution requires a calculation of the following determinant D:

$$D = \begin{vmatrix} \sum X_1^2 & \sum X_1 X_2 \\ \sum X_1 X_2 & \sum X_2^2 \end{vmatrix} = (\sum X_1^2)(\sum X_2^2) - (\sum X_1 X_2)^2 \quad (12.31)$$

from which the coefficients b_1 and b_2 are calculated:

$$b_1 = \begin{vmatrix} \sum YX_1 & \sum X_1 X_2 \\ \sum YX_2 & \sum X_2^2 \end{vmatrix} \div D \qquad (12.32)$$

$$b_2 = \begin{vmatrix} \sum X_1^2 & \sum YX_1 \\ \sum X_1 X_2 & \sum YX_2 \end{vmatrix} \div D . \qquad (12.33)$$

The following *Gaussian coefficients* are needed in the error estimates and these are given by

$$c_{11} = \frac{\sum X_2^2}{D} \qquad c_{22} = \frac{\sum X_1^2}{D} \qquad c_{12} = \frac{-\sum X_1 X_2}{D}. \qquad (12.34)$$

The squared differences between the observed and estimated Y values are summed to give $SS_{res} = \sum (Y - \hat{Y})^2$, which is more readily calculated from

$$SS_{res} = \sum Y^2 - (b_1 \sum X_1 Y + b_2 \sum X_2 Y). \qquad (12.35)$$

From SS_{res} we get the variance

$$s^2 = \frac{SS_{res}}{n - 2} \qquad (12.36)$$

which is used to obtain the needed variances and standard errors calculated as follows:

$$V(b_1) = c_{11}s^2 \qquad V(b_2) = c_{22}s^2 \qquad (12.37)$$

$$SE(b_1) = \sqrt{V(b_1)} \qquad SE(b_2) = \sqrt{V(b_2)}. \qquad (12.38)$$

It is seen that the procedure for nonlinear curve fitting requires extensive computation that is almost always done on a computer. The examples in Chapter 11 used the above procedure at each cycle that produced the data array. The iteration stops when the changes in coefficients b_1 and b_2 become sufficiently small. At that point in the process, the standard errors are those given in Equations 12.38 at this last turn of the cycle.

12.11 Sample size calculations

In numerous applications throughout this book (and several in this chapter) we encountered situations in which a standard error or a confidence interval was calculated. It is clear that the size of the sample is a most important factor in narrowing a confidence interval. Some guidance on sample size is therefore in order to aid planning and executing experiments. If one wishes to test the difference in two populations by sampling from each, the use of very small sample sizes will almost always show that the difference is not significant, even if a difference really exists. This is called a type 2 error or an error due to low power. (A type 1 error occurs when we attribute a significant difference and there is none.) Loosely speaking, statistical power is the ability to detect a difference in cases in which the difference really exists. The power, which is expressed usually as a percentage, e.g., 80% power or 90%, expresses the probability of detecting a significant difference when there is a real difference. Accordingly, we desire sufficient power in our tests; very often 80 or 90% power is used in drug studies. Sometimes certain limitations on the number of subjects force us to lower the power, but when it is possible to do so the sample size (hence, power) should be as large as is practical. The importance is revealed in the several formulas and examples given below which deal with different kinds of statistical tests.

Single proportion

To detect a difference between a test proportion p_1 and a standard proportion, p_0, the sample size is calculated from the equation

$$n = \left\{ \frac{Z_\alpha\sqrt{p_0(1-p_0)} - Z_\beta\sqrt{p_1(1-p_1)}}{p_1 - p_0} \right\}^2 \qquad (12.39)$$

where Z_α = 1.96 (for 95% confidence) and Z_β is one of the following: −1.28 (90% power), −0.84 (80% power) or −0.525 (70% power). Note that Z_α is the two-tailed value from the standard normal curve and Z_β is the lower one-tailed z-value selected for the desired power.

> **Example.** Suppose it is well known that 30% of the residents of a certain community experience allergy symptoms each year. A new preventive inoculation is developed, and it is desired to show that its use can reduce this proportion to 10%. Thus, p_0 = 0.30 and p_1 = 0.10. We use Z_α = 1.96 and Z_β = −0.84 (80% power). Calculation with Equation 12.39 yields n = 33.07; therefore, at least 34 subjects should be tested.

Two proportions

When both control and treatment groups are sampled, and the respective proportions are p_c and p_i, the needed sample size of *each group* to show a difference is the number n calculated from

$$n = \left\{ \frac{Z_\alpha\sqrt{2p_c(1-p_c)} - Z_\beta\sqrt{p_i(1-p_i) + p_c(1-p_c)}}{p_c - p_i} \right\}^2 \qquad (12.40)$$

> **Example.** Suppose it is known that shock occurs in 15% of patients who get a certain infection. A new treatment is said to reduce this proportion to 5%. Studies in both a control and an experimental group are now to be undertaken. These values, p_c = 0.15 and p_i = 0.05, are anticipated. We use the values Z_α = 1.96 and Z_β = −0.84 (80% power) and calculate the number in each group from Equation 12.40; this yields n = 179.9. Thus, 180 patients *in each group* should be tested.

Two means

When two groups are sampled with the aim of detecting a difference in their means, $\mu_1 - \mu_2$, the sample size of each group is calculated from

$$n = 2\left[\frac{(Z_\alpha - Z_\beta)\sigma}{\mu_1 - \mu_2}\right]^2 \tag{12.41}$$

Example. Locomotive behavior in mice is to be studied in a control group and in a group that receives a stimulating drug. Typical scores in this test (in controls) are 200 with a standard deviation of 60. It is anticipated that the scores in the treated group may rise to approximately 250. Using 90% power and the 95% level of significance, we insert $Z_\alpha = 1.96$ and $Z_\beta = -1.28$ into Equation 12.41. This yields $n = 30.23$; thus, 31 are needed in each group. Examination of Equation 12.41 shows that larger differences in the expected means leads to smaller values of n. In other words, detecting small differences requires large sample sizes.

Sample mean

When the mean of a sample (μ_1) is to be compared to a *standard value* (μ_0) the number to be sampled in order to show a significant difference is calculated from

$$n = \left[\frac{(Z_\alpha - Z_\beta)\sigma}{\mu_1 - \mu_0}\right]^2 \tag{12.42}$$

where σ is an estimate of the population standard deviation. Note the difference between this value of n and that when two populations are sampled. The number in this case is half of that which is required when two groups are sampled.

CHAPTER 12

References

Cochran, W.G. Appendix to a paper by F. Tattersfield and J.T. Martin, *Ann. Appl. Biol.* 25:426–429, 1938.

Fieller, E.C. A fundamental formula in the statistics of biological assay, and some applications. *Quart. J. Pharm.* 17:117–123, 1944.

Finney, D.J. *Statistical Methods in Biological Assay,* 2nd ed. London, Charles Griffin and Co. Ltd., 1964.

Computer Software

Information regarding the purchase of the companion software package may be obtained by writing the McCary Group:

The McCary Group
P.O. Box 7105
Elkins Park, PA 19027

jmccary@mccarygroup.com
Website: www.mccarygroup.com

Appendix

Table A-1. Common Logarithms

n	0	1	2	3	4	5	6	7	8	9
1.0	0.0000	0.0043	0.0086	0.0128	0.0170	0.0212	0.0253	0.0294	0.0334	0.0374
1.1	0.0414	0.0453	0.0492	0.0531	0.0569	0.0607	0.0645	0.0682	0.0719	0.0755
1.2	0.0792	0.0828	0.0864	0.0899	0.0934	0.0969	0.1004	0.1038	0.1072	0.1106
1.3	0.1139	0.1173	0.1206	0.1239	0.1271	0.1303	0.1335	0.1367	0.1399	0.1430
1.4	0.1461	0.1492	0.1523	0.1553	0.1584	0.1614	0.1644	0.1673	0.1703	0.1732
1.5	0.1761	0.1790	0.1818	0.1847	0.1875	0.1903	0.1931	0.1959	0.1987	0.2014
1.6	0.2041	0.2068	0.2095	0.2122	0.2148	0.2175	0.2201	0.2227	0.2253	0.2279
1.7	0.2304	0.2330	0.2355	0.2380	0.2405	0.2430	0.2455	0.2480	0.2504	0.2529
1.8	0.2553	0.2577	0.2601	0.2625	0.2648	0.2672	0.2695	0.2718	0.2742	0.2765
1.9	0.2788	0.2810	0.2833	0.2856	0.2878	0.2900	0.2923	0.2945	0.2967	0.2989
2.0	0.3010	0.3032	0.3054	0.3075	0.3096	0.3118	0.3139	0.3160	0.3181	0.3201
2.1	0.3222	0.3243	0.3263	0.3284	0.3304	0.3324	0.3345	0.3365	0.3385	0.3404
2.2	0.3424	0.3444	0.3464	0.3483	0.3502	0.3522	0.3541	0.3560	0.3579	0.3598
2.3	0.3617	0.3636	0.3655	0.3674	0.3692	0.3711	0.3729	0.3747	0.3766	0.3784
2.4	0.3802	0.3820	0.3838	0.3856	0.3874	0.3892	0.3909	0.3927	0.3945	0.3962
2.5	0.3979	0.3997	0.4014	0.4031	0.4048	0.4065	0.4082	0.4099	0.4116	0.4133
2.6	0.4150	0.4166	0.4183	0.4200	0.4216	0.4232	0.4249	0.4265	0.4281	0.4298
2.7	0.4314	0.4330	0.4346	0.4362	0.4378	0.4393	0.4409	0.4425	0.0440	0.4456
2.8	0.4472	0.4487	0.4502	0.4518	0.4533	0.4548	0.4564	0.4579	0.4594	0.4609
2.9	0.4624	0.4639	0.4654	0.4669	0.4683	0.4698	0.4713	0.4728	0.4742	0.4757
3.0	0.4771	0.4786	0.4800	0.4814	0.4829	0.4843	0.4857	0.4871	0.4886	0.4900
3.1	0.4914	0.4928	0.4942	0.4955	0.4969	0.4983	0.4997	0.5011	0.5024	0.5038
3.2	0.5051	0.5065	0.5079	0.5092	0.5105	0.5119	0.5132	0.5145	0.5159	0.5172
3.3	0.5185	0.5198	0.5211	0.5224	0.5237	0.5250	0.5263	0.5276	0.5289	0.5302
3.4	0.5315	0.5328	0.5340	0.5353	0.5366	0.5378	0.5391	0.5403	0.5416	0.5428

continued

Table A-1. (Continued) Common Logarithms

n	0	1	2	3	4	5	6	7	8	9
3.5	0.5441	0.5453	0.5465	0.5478	0.5490	0.5502	0.5514	0.5527	0.5539	0.5551
3.6	0.5563	0.5575	0.5587	0.5599	0.5611	0.5623	0.5635	0.5647	0.5638	0.5670
3.7	0.5682	0.5694	0.5705	0.5717	0.5729	0.5740	0.5752	0.5763	0.5775	0.5786
3.8	0.5798	0.5809	0.5821	0.5832	0.5843	0.5855	0.5866	0.5877	0.5888	0.5899
3.9	0.5911	0.5922	0.5933	0.5944	0.5955	0.5966	0.5977	0.5988	0.5999	0.6010
4.0	0.6021	0.6031	0.6042	0.6053	0.6064	0.6075	0.6085	0.6096	0.6107	0.6117
4.1	0.6128	0.6138	0.6149	0.6160	0.6170	0.6180	0.6191	0.6201	0.6212	0.6222
4.2	0.6232	0.6243	0.6253	0.6263	0.6274	0.6284	0.6294	0.6304	0.6314	0.6325
4.3	0.6335	0.6345	0.6355	0.6365	0.6375	0.6385	0.6395	0.6405	0.6415	0.6425
4.4	0.6435	0.6444	0.6454	0.6464	0.6474	0.6484	0.6493	0.6503	0.6513	0.6522
4.5	0.6532	0.6542	0.6551	0.6561	0.6571	0.6580	0.6590	0.6599	0.6609	0.6618
4.6	0.6628	0.6637	0.6646	0.6656	0.6665	0.6675	0.6684	0.6693	0.6702	0.6712
4.7	0.6721	0.6730	0.6739	0.6749	0.6758	0.6767	0.6776	0.6785	0.6794	0.6803
4.8	0.6812	0.6821	0.6830	0.6839	0.6848	0.6857	0.6866	0.6875	0.6884	0.6893
4.9	0.6902	0.6911	0.6920	0.6928	0.6937	0.6946	0.6955	0.6964	0.6972	0.6981
5.0	0.6990	0.6998	0.7007	0.7016	0.7024	0.7033	0.7042	0.7050	0.7059	0.7067
5.1	0.7076	0.7084	0.7093	0.7101	0.7110	0.7118	0.7126	0.7135	0.7143	0.7152
5.2	0.7160	0.7168	0.7177	0.7185	0.7193	0.7202	0.7210	0.7218	0.7226	0.7235
5.3	0.7243	0.7251	0.7259	0.7267	0.7275	0.7284	0.7292	0.7300	0.7308	0.7316
5.4	0.7324	0.7332	0.7340	0.7348	0.7356	0.7364	0.7372	0.7380	0.7388	0.7396
5.5	0.7404	0.7412	0.7419	0.7427	0.7435	0.7443	0.7451	0.7459	0.7466	0.7474
5.6	0.7482	0.7490	0.7497	0.7505	0.7513	0.7520	0.7528	0.7536	0.7543	0.7551
5.7	0.7559	0.7566	0.7574	0.7582	0.7589	0.7597	0.7604	0.7612	0.7619	0.7627
5.8	0.7634	0.7642	0.7649	0.7657	0.7664	0.7672	0.7679	0.7686	0.7694	0.7701
5.9	0.7709	0.7716	0.7723	0.7731	0.7738	0.7745	0.7752	0.7760	0.7767	0.7774
6.0	0.7782	0.7789	0.7796	0.7803	0.7810	0.7818	0.7825	0.7832	0.7839	0.7846
6.1	0.7853	0.7860	0.7868	0.7875	0.7882	0.7889	0.7896	0.7903	0.7910	0.7917
6.2	0.7924	0.7931	0.7938	0.7945	0.7952	0.7959	0.7966	0.7973	0.7980	0.7987
6.3	0.7993	0.8000	0.8007	0.8014	0.8021	0.8028	0.8035	0.8041	0.8048	0.8055
6.4	0.8062	0.8069	0.8075	0.8082	0.8089	0.8096	0.8102	0.8109	0.8116	0.8122
6.5	0.8129	0.8136	0.8142	0.8149	0.8156	0.8162	0.8169	0.8176	0.8182	0.8189
6.6	0.8195	0.8202	0.8209	0.8215	0.8222	0.8228	0.8235	0.8241	0.8248	0.8254
6.7	0.8261	0.8267	0.8274	0.8280	0.8287	0.8293	0.8299	0.8306	0.8312	0.8319
6.8	0.8325	0.8331	0.8338	0.8344	0.8351	0.8357	0.8363	0.8370	0.8376	0.8382
6.9	0.8388	0.8395	0.8401	0.8407	0.8414	0.8420	0.8426	0.8432	0.8439	0.8445

Table A-1. (Continued) Common Logarithms

n	0	1	2	3	4	5	6	7	8	9
7.0	0.8451	0.8457	0.8463	0.8470	0.8476	0.8482	0.8488	0.8494	0.8500	0.8506
7.1	0.8513	0.8519	0.8525	0.8531	0.8537	0.8543	0.8549	0.8555	0.8561	0.8567
7.2	0.8573	0.8579	0.8585	0.8591	0.8597	0.8603	0.8609	0.8615	0.8621	0.8627
7.3	0.8633	0.8639	0.8645	0.8651	0.8657	0.8663	0.8669	0.8675	0.8681	0.8686
7.4	0.8692	0.8698	0.8704	0.8710	0.8716	0.8722	0.8727	0.8733	0.8739	0.8745
7.5	0.8751	0.8756	0.8762	0.8768	0.8774	0.8779	0.8785	0.8791	0.8797	0.8802
7.6	0.8808	0.8814	0.8820	0.8825	0.8831	0.8837	0.8842	0.8848	0.8854	0.8859
7.7	0.8865	0.8871	0.8876	0.8882	0.8887	0.8893	0.8899	0.8904	0.8910	0.8915
7.8	0.8921	0.8927	0.8932	0.8938	0.8943	0.8949	0.8954	0.8960	0.8965	0.8971
7.9	0.8976	0.8982	0.8987	0.8993	0.8998	0.9004	0.9009	0.9015	0.9020	0.9025
8.0	0.9031	0.9036	0.9042	0.9047	0.9053	0.9058	0.9063	0.9069	0.9074	0.9079
8.1	0.9085	0.9090	0.9096	0.9101	0.9106	0.9112	0.9117	0.9122	0.9128	0.9133
8.2	0.9138	0.9143	0.9149	0.9154	0.9159	0.9165	0.9170	0.9175	0.9180	0.9186
8.3	0.9191	0.9196	0.9201	0.9206	0.9212	0.9217	0.9222	0.9227	0.9232	0.9238
8.4	0.2943	0.9248	0.9253	0.9258	0.9263	0.9269	0.9274	0.9279	0.9284	0.9289
8.5	0.9294	0.9299	0.9304	0.9309	0.9315	0.9320	0.9325	0.9330	0.9335	0.9340
8.6	0.9345	0.9350	0.9355	0.9360	0.9365	0.9370	0.9375	0.9380	0.9385	0.9390
8.7	0.9395	0.9400	0.9405	0.9410	0.9415	0.9420	0.9425	0.9430	0.9435	0.9440
8.8	0.9445	0.9450	0.9455	0.9460	0.9465	0.9469	0.9474	0.9479	0.9484	0.9489
8.9	0.9494	0.9499	0.9504	0.9509	0.9513	0.9518	0.9523	0.9528	0.9533	0.9538
9.0	0.9542	0.9547	0.9552	0.9557	0.9562	0.9566	0.9571	0.9576	0.9581	0.9586
9.1	0.9590	0.9595	0.9600	0.9605	0.9609	0.9614	0.9619	0.9624	0.9628	0.9633
9.2	0.9638	0.9643	0.9647	0.9652	0.9657	0.9661	0.9666	0.9671	0.9675	0.9680
9.3	0.9685	0.9689	0.9694	0.9699	0.9703	0.9708	0.9713	0.9717	0.9722	0.9727
9.4	0.9731	0.9736	0.9741	0.9745	0.9750	0.9754	0.9759	0.9763	0.9768	0.9773
9.5	0.9777	0.9782	0.9786	0.9791	0.9795	0.9800	0.9805	0.9809	0.9814	0.9818
9.6	0.9823	0.9827	0.9832	0.9836	0.9841	0.9845	0.9850	0.9854	0.9859	0.9863
9.7	0.9868	0.9872	0.9877	0.9881	0.9886	0.9890	0.9894	0.9899	0.9903	0.9908
9.8	0.9912	0.9917	0.9921	0.9926	0.9930	0.9934	0.9939	0.9943	0.9948	0.9952
9.9	0.9956	0.9661	0.9965	0.996	0.9974	0.9978	0.9983	0.9987	0.9991	0.9996

Reprinted from Tallarida, R.J. and Murray, R.B., *Manual of Pharmacologic Calculations with Computer Programs*, 2nd ed 1987. By permission of Springer-Verlag, New York.

Table A-2 . Natural Logarithms

x	$\ln x$	x	$\ln x$	x	$\ln x$
0.1	7.6974–10	3.6	1.2809	7.1	1.9601
0.2	8.3906–10	3.7	1.3083	7.2	1.9741
0.3	8.7960–10	3.8	1.3350	7.3	1.9879
0.4	9.0837–10	3.9	1.3610	7.4	2.0015
0.5	9.3069–10	4.0	1.3863	7.5	2.0149
0.6	9.4892–10	4.1	1.4110	7.6	2.0281
0.7	9.6433–10	4.2	1.4351	7.7	2.0412
0.8	9.7769–10	4.3	1.4586	7.8	2.0541
0.9	9.8946–10	4.4	1.4816	7.9	2.0669
1.0	0.0000	4.5	1.5041	8.0	2.0794
1.1	0.0953	4.6	1.5261	8.1	2.0919
1.2	0.1823	4.7	1.5476	8.2	2.1041
1.3	0.2624	4.8	1.5686	8.3	2.1163
1.4	0.3365	4.9	1.5892	8.4	2.1182
1.5	0.4055	5.0	1.6094	8.5	2.1401
1.6	0.4700	5.1	1.6292	8.6	2.1518
1.7	0.5306	5.2	1.6487	8.7	2.1633
1.8	0.5878	5.3	1.6677	8.8	2.1748
1.9	0.6419	5.4	1.6864	8.9	2.1861
2.0	0.6931	5.5	1.7047	9.0	2.1972
2.1	0.7419	5.6	1.7228	9.1	2.2083
2.2	0.7885	5.7	1.7405	9.2	2.2192
2.3	0.8329	5.8	1.7579	9.3	2.2300
2.4	0.8755	5.9	1.7750	9.4	2.2407
2.5	0.9163	6.0	1.7918	9.5	2.2513
2.6	0.9555	6.1	1.8083	9.6	2.2618
2.7	0.9933	6.2	1.8245	9.7	2.2721
2.8	1.0296	6.3	1.8405	9.8	2.2824
2.9	1.0647	6.4	1.8563	9.9	2.2925
3.0	1.0986	6.5	1.8718	10	2.3026
3.1	1.1314	6.6	1.8871	11	2.3979
3.2	1.1632	6.7	1.9021	12	2.4849
3.3	1.1939	6.8	1.9169	13	2.5649
3.4	1.2238	6.9	1.9315	14	2.6391
3.5	1.2528	7.0	1.9459	15	2.7081

Table A-2 (Continued) . Natural Logarithms

x	$\ln x$	x	$\ln x$	x	$\ln x$
16	2.7726	45	3.8067	90	4.4998
17	2.8322	50	3.9120	95	4.5539
18	2.8904	55	4.0073	100	4.6052
19	2.9444	60	4.0943		
20	2.9957	65	4.1744		
25	3.2189	70	4.2485		
30	3.4012	75	4.3175		
35	3.5553	80	4.3820		
40	3.6889	85	4.4427		

Reprinted from Tallarida, R.J. and Murray, R.B., *Manual of Pharmacologic Calculations with Computer Programs*, 2nd ed 1987. By permission of Springer-Verlag, New York.

Table A-3. Powers of e: $\exp(x)$ and $\exp(-x)$

x	e^x	e^{-x}	x	e^x	e^{-x}
0.00	1.00000	1.00000	1.40	4.05519	0.24659
0.01	1.01005	0.99004	1.50	4.48168	0.22313
0.02	1.02020	0.98019	1.60	4.95302	0.20189
0.03	1.03045	0.97044	1.70	5.47394	0.18268
0.04	1.04081	0.96078	1.80	6.04964	0.16529
0.05	1.05127	0.95122	1.90	6.68589	0.14956
0.06	1.06183	0.94176	2.00	7.38905	0.13533
0.07	1.07250	0.93239	2.10	8.16616	0.12245
0.08	1.08328	0.92311	2.20	9.02500	0.11080
0.09	1.09417	0.91393	2.30	9.97417	0.10025
0.10	1.10517	0.90483	2.40	11.02316	0.09071
0.11	1.11628	0.89583	2.50	12.18248	0.08208
0.12	1.12750	0.88692	2.60	13.46372	0.07427
0.13	1.13883	0.87810	2.70	14.87971	0.06720
0.14	1.15027	0.86936	2.80	16.44463	0.06081
0.15	1.16183	0.86071	2.90	18.17412	0.05502
0.16	1.17351	0.85214	3.00	20.08551	0.04978
0.17	1.18530	0.84366	3.50	33.11545	0.03020
0.18	1.19722	0.83527	4.00	54.95815	0.01832
0.19	1.20925	0.82696	4.50	90.01713	0.01111
0.20	1.22140	0.81873	5.00	148.41316	0.00674
0.30	1.34985	0.74081	5.50	244.69193	0.00409
0.40	1.49182	0.67032	6.00	403.42879	0.00248
0.50	1.64872	0.60653	6.50	665.14163	0.00150
0.60	1.82211	0.54881	7.00	1096.63316	0.00091
0.70	2.01375	0.49658	7.50	1808.04241	0.00055
0.80	2.22554	0.44932	8.00	2980.95799	0.00034
0.90	2.45960	0.40656	8.50	4914.76884	0.00020
1.00	2.71828	0.36787	9.00	8103.08398	0.00012
1.10	3.00416	0.33287	9.50	13359.72683	0.00007
1.20	3.32011	0.30119	10.00	22026.46579	0.00005
1.30	3.66929	0.27253			

Reprinted from Tallarida, R.J. and Murray, R.B., *Manual of Pharmacologic Calculations with Computer Programs*, 2nd ed 1987. By permission of Springer-Verlag, New York.

Table A-4. Squares and Square Roots

n	n^2	$\sqrt{n}$	$\sqrt{10n}$	n	n^2	$\sqrt{n}$	$\sqrt{10n}$
1	1	1.000	3.162	36	1296	6.000	18.974
2	4	1.414	4.472	37	1369	6.083	19.235
3	9	1.732	5.477	38	1444	6.164	19.494
4	16	2.000	6.325	39	1521	6.245	19.748
5	25	2.236	7.071	40	1600	6.325	20.000
6	36	2.449	7.746	41	1681	6.403	20.248
7	49	2.646	8.367	42	1764	6.481	20.494
8	64	2.828	8.944	43	1849	6.557	20.736
9	81	3.000	9.487	44	1936	6.633	20.976
10	100	3.162	10.000	45	2025	6.708	21.213
11	121	3.317	10.488	46	2116	6.782	21.448
12	144	3.464	10.954	47	2209	6.856	21.679
13	169	3.606	11.042	48	2304	6.928	21.909
14	196	3.742	11.832	49	2401	7.000	22.136
15	225	3.873	12.247	50	2500	7.071	22.361
16	256	4.000	12.649	51	2601	7.141	22.583
17	289	4.123	13.038	52	2704	7.211	22.804
18	324	4.243	13.416	53	2809	7.280	23.022
19	361	4.359	13.784	54	2916	7.348	23.238
20	400	4.472	14.142	55	3025	7.416	23.452
21	441	4.583	14.491	56	3136	7.483	23.664
22	484	4.690	14.832	57	3249	7.550	23.875
23	529	4.796	15.166	58	3364	7.616	24.083
24	576	4.899	15.492	59	3481	7.681	24.290
25	625	5.000	15.811	60	3600	7.746	24.495
26	676	5.099	16.125	61	3721	7.810	24.698
27	729	5.196	16.432	62	3844	7.874	24.900
28	784	5.292	16.733	63	3969	7.937	25.100
29	841	5.385	17.029	64	4096	8.000	25.298
30	900	5.477	17.321	65	4225	8.062	25.495
31	961	5.568	17.607	66	4056	8.124	25.690
32	1024	5.657	17.889	67	4489	8.185	25.884
33	1089	5.745	18.166	68	4624	8.246	26.077
34	1156	5.831	18.439	69	4761	8.307	26.268
35	1225	5.916	18.708	70	4900	8.367	26.458

continued

Table A-4. (Continued) Squares and Square Roots

n	n^2	$\sqrt{n}$	$\sqrt{10n}$	n	n^2	$\sqrt{n}$	$\sqrt{10n}$
71	5041	8.426	26.646	86	7396	9.274	29.326
72	5184	8.485	26.833	87	7569	9.327	29.496
73	5329	8.544	27.019	88	7744	9.381	29.665
74	5476	8.602	27.203	89	7921	9.434	29.833
75	5625	8.660	27.386	90	8100	9.487	30.000
76	5776	8.718	27.568	91	8281	9.539	30.166
77	5929	8.775	27.749	92	8464	9.592	30.332
78	6084	8.832	27.928	93	8649	9.644	30.496
79	6241	8.888	28.107	94	8836	9.695	30.659
80	6400	8.944	28.284	95	9025	9.747	30.822
81	6561	9.000	28.460	96	9216	9.798	30.984
82	6724	9.055	28.636	97	9409	9.849	31.145
83	6889	9.110	28.810	98	9604	9.899	31.305
84	7056	9.165	28.983	99	9801	9.950	31.464
85	7225	9.220	29.155	100	10000	10.000	31.623

Reprinted from Tallarida, R.J. and Murray, R.B., *Manual of Pharmacologic Calculations with Computer Programs*, 2nd ed 1987. By permission of Springer-Verlag, New York.

Table A-5. Areas Under the Standard Normal Curve

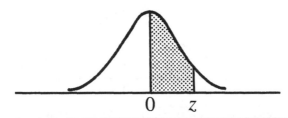

z	0.00	0.01	0.02	0.03	0.04	0.05	0.06	0.07	0.08	0.09
0.0	0.0000	0.0040	0.0080	0.0120	0.0160	0.0199	0.0239	0.0279	0.0319	0.0359
0.1	0.0398	0.0438	0.0478	0.0517	0.0557	0.0596	0.0636	0.0675	0.0714	0.0753
0.2	0.0793	0.0832	0.0871	0.0910	0.0948	0.0987	0.1026	0.1064	0.1103	0.1141
0.3	0.1179	0.1217	0.1255	0.1293	0.1331	0.1368	0.1406	0.1443	0.1480	0.1517
0.4	0.1554	0.1591	0.1628	0.1664	0.1700	0.1736	0.1772	0.1808	0.1844	0.1879
0.5	0.1915	0.1950	0.1985	0.2019	0.2054	0.2088	0.2123	0.2157	0.2190	0.2224
0.6	0.2257	0.2291	0.2324	0.2357	0.2389	0.2422	0.2454	0.2486	0.2517	0.2549
0.7	0.2580	0.2611	0.2642	0.2673	0.2704	0.2734	0.2764	0.2794	0.2823	0.2852
0.8	0.2881	0.2910	0.2939	0.2967	0.2995	0.3023	0.3051	0.3078	0.3106	0.3133
0.9	0.3159	0.3186	0.3212	0.3238	0.3264	0.3289	0.3315	0.3340	0.3365	0.3389
1.0	0.3413	0.3438	0.3461	0.3485	0.3508	0.3531	0.3554	0.3577	0.3599	0.3621
1.1	0.3643	0.3665	0.3686	0.3708	0.3729	0.3749	0.3770	0.3790	0.3810	0.3830
1.2	0.3849	0.3869	0.3888	0.3907	0.3925	0.3944	0.3962	0.3980	0.3997	0.4015
1.3	0.4032	0.4049	0.4066	0.4082	0.4099	0.4115	0.4131	0.4147	0.4162	0.4177
1.4	0.4192	0.4207	0.4222	0.4236	0.4251	0.4265	0.4279	0.4292	0.4306	0.4319
1.5	0.4332	0.4345	0.4357	0.4370	0.4382	0.4394	0.4406	0.4418	0.4429	0.4441
1.6	0.4452	0.4463	0.4474	0.4484	0.4495	0.4505	0.4515	0.4525	0.4535	0.4545
1.7	0.4554	0.4564	0.4573	0.4582	0.4591	0.4599	0.4608	0.4616	0.4625	0.4633
1.8	0.4641	0.4649	0.4656	0.4664	0.4671	0.4678	0.4686	0.4693	0.4699	0.4706
1.9	0.4713	0.4719	0.4726	0.4732	0.4738	0.4744	0.4750	0.4756	0.4761	0.4767
2.0	0.4772	0.4778	0.4783	0.4788	0.4793	0.4798	0.4803	0.4808	0.4812	0.4817
2.1	0.4821	0.4826	0.4830	0.4834	0.4838	0.4842	0.4846	0.4850	0.4854	0.4857
2.2	0.4861	0.4864	0.4868	0.4871	0.4875	0.4878	0.4881	0.4884	0.4887	0.4890
2.3	0.4893	0.4896	0.4898	0.4901	0.4904	0.4906	0.4909	0.4911	0.4913	0.4916
2.4	0.4918	0.4920	0.4922	0.4925	0.4927	0.4929	0.4931	0.4932	0.4934	0.4936
2.5	0.4938	0.4940	0.4941	0.4943	0.4945	0.4946	0.4948	0.4949	0.4951	0.4952
2.6	0.4953	0.4955	0.4956	0.4957	0.4959	0.4960	0.4961	0.4962	0.4963	0.4964
2.7	0.4965	0.4966	0.4967	0.4968	0.4969	0.4970	0.4971	0.4972	0.4973	0.4974
2.8	0.4974	0.4975	0.4976	0.4977	0.4977	0.4978	0.4979	0.4979	0.4980	0.4981
2.9	0.4981	0.4982	0.4982	0.4983	0.4984	0.4984	0.4985	0.4985	0.4986	0.4986
3.0	0.4987	0.4987	0.4987	0.4988	0.4988	0.4989	0.4989	0.4989	0.4990	0.4990

Reprinted from Tallarida, R.J. and Murray, R.B., *Manual of Pharmacologic Calculations with Computer Programs*, 2nd ed 1987. By permission of Springer-Verlag, New York.

Table A-6. *t* Distribution

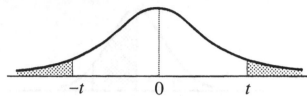

deg. freedom, v	90% ($P = 0.1$)	95% ($P = 0.05$)	99% ($P = 0.01$)
1	6.314	12.706	63.657
2	2.920	4.303	9.925
3	2.353	3.182	5.841
4	2.132	2.776	4.604
5	2.015	2.571	4.032
6	1.943	2.447	3.707
7	1.895	2.365	3.499
8	1.860	2.306	3.355
9	1.833	2.262	3.250
10	1.812	2.228	3.169
11	1.796	2.201	3.106
12	1.782	2.179	3.055
13	1.771	2.160	3.012
14	1.761	2.145	2.977
15	1.753	2.131	2.947
16	1.746	2.120	2.921
17	1.740	2.110	2.898
18	1.734	2.101	2.878
19	1,729	2.093	2.861
20	1.725	2.086	2.845
21	1.721	2.080	2.831
22	1.717	2.074	2.819
23	1.714	2.069	2.807
24	1.711	2.064	2.797
25	1.708	2.060	2.787
26	1.706	2.056	2.779
27	1.703	2.052	2.771
28	1.701	2.048	2.763
29	1.699	2.045	2.756
inf.	1.645	1.960	2.576

Reprinted from Tallarida, R.J. and Murray, R.B., *Manual of Pharmacologic Calculations with Computer Programs*, 2nd ed 1987. By permission of Springer-Verlag, New York.

Table A-7. Chi Square

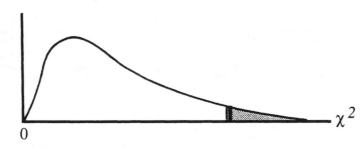

v	0.05	0.025	0.01	0.005
1	3.841	5.024	6.635	7.879
2	5.991	7.378	9.210	10.597
3	7.815	9.348	11.345	12.838
4	9.488	11.143	13.277	14.860
5	11.070	12.832	15.086	16.750
6	12.592	14.449	16.812	18.548
7	14.067	16.013	18.475	20.278
8	15.507	17.535	20.090	21.955
9	16.919	19.023	21.666	23.589
10	18.307	20.483	23.209	25.188
11	19.675	21.920	24.725	26.757
12	21.026	23.337	26.217	28.300
13	22.362	24.736	27.688	29.819
14	23.685	26.119	29.141	31.319
15	24.996	27.488	30.578	32.801
16	26.296	28.845	32.000	34.267
17	27.587	30.191	33.409	35.718
18	28.869	31.526	34.805	37.156
19	30.144	32.852	36.191	38.582
20	31.410	34.170	37.566	39.997
21	32.671	35.479	38.932	41.401
22	33.924	36.781	40.289	42.796
23	35.172	38.076	41.638	44.101
24	36.415	39.364	42.980	45.558
25	37.652	40.646	44.314	46.928
26	38.885	41.923	45.642	48.290
27	40.113	43.194	46.963	49.645

continued

Table A-7. (Continued) Chi Square

ν	0.05	0.025	0.01	0.005
28	41.337	44.461	48.278	50.993
29	42.257	45.722	49.588	52.336
30	43.773	46.979	50.892	53.672

Table A-8. Probit Transformation

Probit	Proportion	Probit	Proportion	Probit	Proportion
1.00	0.00003167	1.41	0.00016534	1.82	0.00073638
1.01	0.00003304	1.42	0.00017180	1.83	0.00076219
1.02	0.00003446	1.43	0.00017849	1.84	0.00078885
1.03	0.00003594	1.44	0.00018543	1.85	0.00081635
1.04	0.00003747	1.45	0.00019262	1.86	0.00084474
1.05	0.00003908	1.46	0.00020006	1.87	0.00087403
1.06	0.00004074	1.47	0.00020778	1.88	0.00090426
1.07	0.00004247	1.48	0.00021577	1.89	0.00093544
1.08	0.00004427	1.49	0.00022405	1.90	0.00096760
1.09	0.00004615	1.50	0.00023263	1.91	0.00100078
1.10	0.00004810	1.51	0.00024151	1.92	0.00103500
1.11	0.00005012	1.52	0.00025071	1.93	0.00107029
1.12	0.00005223	1.53	0.00026063	1.94	0.00110669
1.13	0.00005442	1.54	0.00027009	1.95	0.00114421
1.14	0.00005669	1.55	0.00028029	1.96	0.00118289
1.15	0.00005906	1.56	0.00029086	1.97	0.00122277
1.16	0.00006152	1.57	0.00030179	1.98	0.00126387
1.17	0.00006407	1.58	0.00031311	1.99	0.00130624
1.18	0.00006673	1.59	0.00032481	2.00	0.00134990
1.19	0.00006948	1.60	0.00033693	2.01	0.00139489
1.20	0.00007235	1.61	0.00034946	2.02	0.00144124
1.21	0.00007532	1.62	0.00036243	2.03	0.00148900
1.22	0.00007841	1.63	0.00037584	2.04	0.00153820
1.23	0.00008162	1.64	0.00038971	2.05	0.00158887
1.24	0.00008496	1.65	0.00040406	2.06	0.00164106
1.25	0.00008842	1.66	0.00041889	2.07	0.00169481
1.26	0.00009201	1.67	0.00043423	2.08	0.00175016
1.27	0.00009574	1.68	0.00045009	2.09	0.00180714
1.28	0.00009961	1.69	0.00046648	2.10	0.00186581
1.29	0.00010363	1.70	0.00048342	2.11	0.00192621
1.30	0.00010780	1.71	0.00050094	2.12	0.00198838
1.31	0.00011213	1.72	0.00051904	2.13	0.00205236
1.32	0.00011662	1.73	0.00053774	2.14	0.00211821
1.33	0.00012128	1.74	0.00055706	2.15	0.00218596
1.34	0.00012611	1.75	0.00057703	2.16	0.00225568
1.35	0.00013112	1.76	0.00059765	2.17	0.00232740
1.36	0.00013632	1.77	0.00061895	2.18	0.00240118
1.37	0.00014171	1.78	0.00064095	2.19	0.00247708
1.38	0.00014730	1.79	0.00066367	2.20	0.00255513
1.39	0.00015310	1.80	0.00068714	2.21	0.00263540
1.40	0.00015911	1.81	0.00071136	2.22	0.00271794

continued

Table A-8. (Continued) Probit Transformation

Probit	Proportion	Probit	Proportion	Probit	Proportion
2.23	0.00280281	2.66	0.00964187	3.09	0.02806661
2.24	0.00289007	2.67	0.00990308	3.10	0.02871656
2.25	0.00297976	2.68	0.01017044	3.11	0.02937898
2.26	0.00307196	2.69	0.01044408	3.12	0.03005404
2.27	0.00316672	2.70	0.01072411	3.13	0.03074191
2.28	0.00326410	2.71	0.01101066	3.14	0.03144276
2.29	0.00336416	2.72	0.01130384	3.15	0.03215678
2.30	0.00346697	2.73	0.01160379	3.16	0.03288412
2.31	0.00357260	2.74	0.01191063	3.17	0.03362497
2.32	0.00368111	2.75	0.01222447	3.18	0.03437950
2.33	0.00379256	2.76	0.01254546	3.19	0.03514789
2.34	0.00390703	2.77	0.01287372	3.20	0.03593032
2.35	0.00402459	2.78	0.01320938	3.21	0.03672696
2.36	0.00414530	2.79	0.01355258	3.22	0.03753798
2.37	0.00426924	2.80	0.01390345	3.23	0.03836357
2.38	0.00439649	2.81	0.01426212	3.24	0.03920390
2.39	0.00452711	2.82	0.01462873	3.25	0.04005916
2.40	0.00466119	2.83	0.01500342	3.26	0.04092951
2.41	0.00479880	2.84	0.01538634	3.27	0.04181514
2.42	0.00494002	2.85	0.01577761	3.28	0.04271622
2.43	0.00508493	2.86	0.01617738	3.29	0.04363294
2.44	0.00523361	2.87	0.01658581	3.30	0.04456546
2.45	0.00538615	2.88	0.01700302	3.31	0.04551398
2.46	0.00554262	2.89	0.01742918	3.32	0.04647866
2.47	0.00570313	2.90	0.01786442	3.33	0.04745968
2.48	0.00586774	2.91	0.01830890	3.34	0.04845723
2.49	0.00603656	2.92	0.01876277	3.35	0.04947147
2.50	0.00620967	2.93	0.01922617	3.36	0.05050258
2.51	0.00638715	2.94	0.01969927	3.37	0.05155075
2.52	0.00656912	2.95	0.02018222	3.38	0.05261614
2.53	0.00675565	2.96	0.02067516	3.39	0.05369893
2.54	0.00694685	2.97	0.02117827	3.40	0.05479929
2.55	0.00714281	2.98	0.02169169	3.41	0.05591740
2.56	0.00734363	2.99	0.02221559	3.42	0.05705343
2.57	0.00754941	3.00	0.02275013	3.43	0.05820756
2.58	0.00776025	3.01	0.02329547	3.44	0.05937994
2.59	0.00797626	3.02	0.02385176	3.45	0.06057076
2.60	0.00819754	3.03	0.02441919	3.46	0.06178018
2.61	0.00842419	3.04	0.02499790	3.47	0.06300836
2.62	0.00865632	3.05	0.02558806	3.48	0.06425549
2.63	0.00889404	3.06	0.02618985	3.49	0.06552171
2.64	0.00913747	3.07	0.02680342	3.50	0.06680720
2.65	0.00938671	3.08	0.02742895	3.51	0.06811212

Table A-8. (Continued) Probit Transformation

Probit	Proportion	Probit	Proportion	Probit	Proportion
3.52	0.06943662	3.93	0.14230965	4.34	0.25462691
3.53	0.07078088	3.94	0.14457230	4.35	0.25784611
3.54	0.07214504	3.95	0.14685906	4.36	0.26108630
3.55	0.07352926	3.96	0.14916995	4.37	0.26434729
3.56	0.07493370	3.97	0.15150500	4.38	0.26762889
3.57	0.07635851	3.98	0.15386423	4.39	0.27093090
3.58	0.07780384	3.99	0.15624765	4.40	0.27425312
3.59	0.07926984	4.00	0.15865525	4.41	0.27759532
3.60	0.08075666	4.01	0.16108706	4.42	0.28095731
3.61	0.08226444	4.02	0.16354306	4.43	0.28433885
3.62	0.08379332	4.03	0.16602325	4.44	0.28773972
3.63	0.08534345	4.04	0.16852761	4.45	0.29115969
3.64	0.08691496	4.05	0.17105613	4.46	0.29459852
3.65	0.08850799	4.06	0.17360878	4.47	0.29805597
3.66	0.09012267	4.07	0.17618554	4.48	0.30153179
3.67	0.09175914	4.08	0.17878638	4.49	0.30502573
3.68	0.09341751	4.09	0.18141125	4.50	0.30853754
3.69	0.09509792	4.10	0.18406013	4.51	0.31206695
3.70	0.09680049	4.11	0.18673294	4.52	0.31561370
3.71	0.09852533	4.12	0.18942965	4.53	0.31917751
3.72	0.10027257	4.13	0.19215020	4.54	0.32275811
3.73	0.10204232	4.14	0.19489452	4.55	0.32635522
3.74	0.10383468	4.15	0.19766254	4.56	0.32996855
3.75	0.10564977	4.16	0.20045419	4.57	0.33359782
3.76	0.10748770	4.17	0.20326939	4.58	0.33724273
3.77	0.10934855	4.18	0.20610805	4.59	0.34090297
3.78	0.11123244	4.19	0.20897009	4.60	0.34457826
3.79	0.11313945	4.20	0.21185540	4.61	0.34826827
3.80	0.11506967	4.21	0.21476388	4.62	0.35197271
3.81	0.11702320	4.22	0.21769544	4.63	0.35569125
3.82	0.11900011	4.23	0.22064995	4.64	0.35942357
3.83	0.12100048	4.24	0.22362729	4.65	0.36316935
3.84	0.12302440	4.25	0.22662735	4.66	0.36692826
3.85	0.12507194	4.26	0.22965000	4.67	0.37069998
3.86	0.12714315	4.27	0.23269509	4.68	0.37448417
3.87	0.12923811	4.28	0.23576250	4.69	0.37828048
3.88	0.13135688	4.29	0.23885207	4.70	0.38208858
3.89	0.13349951	4.30	0.24196365	4.71	0.38590812
3.90	0.13566606	4.31	0.24509709	4.72	0.38973875
3.91	0.13785657	4.32	0.24825223	4.73	0.39358013
3.92	0.14007109	4.33	0.25142890	4.74	0.39743189

continued

Table A-8. (Continued) Probit Transformation

Probit	Proportion	Probit	Proportion	Probit	Proportion
4.75	0.40129367	5.18	0.57142372	5.61	0.72906910
4.76	0.40516513	5.19	0.57534543	5.62	0.73237111
4.77	0.40904588	5.20	0.57925971	5.63	0.73565271
4.78	0.41293558	5.21	0.58316616	5.64	0.73891370
4.79	0.41683384	5.22	0.58706442	5.65	0.74215389
4.80	0.42074029	5.23	0.59095412	5.66	0.74537309
4.81	0.42465457	5.24	0.59483487	5.67	0.74857110
4.82	0.42857628	5.25	0.59870633	5.68	0.75174777
4.83	0.43250507	5.26	0.60256811	5.69	0.75490291
4.84	0.43644054	5.27	0.60641987	5.70	0.75803635
4.85	0.44038231	5.28	0.61026125	5.71	0.76114793
4.86	0.44433000	5.29	0.61409188	5.72	0.76423750
4.87	0.44828321	5.30	0.61791142	5.73	0.76730491
4.88	0.45224157	5.31	0.62171952	5.74	0.77035000
4.89	0.45620469	5.32	0.62551583	5.75	0.77337265
4.90	0.46017216	5.33	0.62930002	5.76	0.77637271
4.91	0.46414361	5.34	0.63307174	5.77	0.77935005
4.92	0.46811863	5.35	0.63683065	5.78	0.78230456
4.93	0.47209683	5.36	0.64057643	5.79	0.78523612
4.94	0.47607782	5.37	0.64403875	5.80	0.78814460
4.95	0.48006119	5.38	0.64802729	5.81	0.79102991
4.96	0.48404656	5.39	0.65173173	5.82	0.79389195
4.97	0.48803353	5.40	0.65542174	5.83	0.79673061
4.98	0.49202169	5.41	0.65909703	5.84	0.79954581
4.99	0.49601064	5.42	0.66275727	5.85	0.80233746
5.00	0.50000000	5.43	0.66640218	5.86	0.80510548
5.01	0.50398936	5.44	0.67003145	5.87	0.80784980
5.02	0.50797831	5.45	0.67364478	5.88	0.81057035
5.03	0.51196647	5.46	0.67724189	5.89	0.81326706
5.04	0.51595344	5.47	0.68082249	5.90	0.81593987
5.05	0.51993881	5.48	0.68438630	5.91	0.81858875
5.06	0.52392218	5.49	0.68793305	5.92	0.82121362
5.07	0.52790317	5.50	0.69146246	5.93	0.82381446
5.08	0.53188137	5.51	0.69497427	5.94	0.82639122
5.09	0.53585639	5.52	0.69846821	5.95	0.82894387
5.10	0.53982784	5.53	0.70194403	5.96	0.83147239
5.11	0.54379531	5.54	0.70540148	5.97	0.83397675
5.12	0.54775843	5.55	0.70884031	5.98	0.83645694
5.13	0.55171679	5.56	0.71226028	5.99	0.83891294
5.14	0.55567000	5.57	0.71566115	6.00	0.84134475
5.15	0.55961769	5.58	0.71904269	6.01	0.84375235
5.16	0.56355946	5.59	0.72240468	6.02	0.84613577
5.17	0.56749493	5.60	0.72574688	6.03	0.84849500

Table A-8. (Continued) Probit Transformation

Probit	Proportion	Probit	Proportion	Probit	Proportion
6.04	0.85083005	6.46	0.92785496	6.88	0.96994596
6.05	0.85314094	6.47	0.92921912	6.89	0.97062102
6.06	0.85542770	6.48	0.93056338	6.90	0.97128344
6.07	0.85769035	6.49	0.93188788	6.91	0.97193339
6.08	0.85992891	6.50	0.93319280	6.92	0.97257105
6.09	0.86214343	6.51	0.93447829	6.93	0.97319658
6.10	0.86433394	6.52	0.93574451	6.94	0.97381016
6.11	0.86650049	6.53	0.93699164	6.95	0.97441194
6.12	0.86864312	6.54	0.93821982	6.96	0.97500210
6.13	0.87076189	6.55	0.93942924	6.97	0.97558081
6.14	0.87285685	6.56	0.94062006	6.98	0.97614824
6.15	0.87492806	6.57	0.94179244	6.99	0.97670453
6.16	0.87697560	6.58	0.94294657	7.00	0.97724987
6.17	0.87899952	6.59	0.94408260	7.01	0.97778441
6.18	0.88099989	6.60	0.94520071	7.02	0.97830831
6.19	0.88297680	6.61	0.94630107	7.03	0.97882173
6.20	0.88493033	6.62	0.94738386	7.04	0.97932484
6.21	0.88686055	6.63	0.94844925	7.05	0.97981778
6.22	0.88876756	6.64	0.94949742	7.06	0.98030073
6.23	0.89065145	6.65	0.95052853	7.07	0.98077383
6.24	0.89251230	6.66	0.95154277	7.08	0.98123723
6.25	0.89435023	6.67	0.95254032	7.09	0.98169110
6.26	0.89616532	6.68	0.95352134	7.10	0.98213558
6.27	0.89795768	6.69	0.95448602	7.11	0.98257082
6.28	0.89972743	6.70	0.95543454	7.12	0.98299698
6.29	0.90147467	6.71	0.95636706	7.13	0.98341419
6.30	0.90319952	6.72	0.95728878	7.14	0.98382262
6.31	0.90490208	6.73	0.95818486	7.15	0.98422239
6.32	0.90658249	6.74	0.95907049	7.16	0.98461367
6.33	0.90824086	6.75	0.95994084	7.17	0.98499658
6.34	0.90987733	6.76	0.96079610	7.18	0.98537127
6.35	0.91149201	6.77	0.96163643	7.19	0.98573788
6.36	0.91308504	6.78	0.96246202	7.20	0.98609655
6.37	0.91465655	6.79	0.96327304	7.21	0.98644742
6.38	0.91620668	6.80	0.96406968	7.22	0.98679062
6.39	0.91773556	6.81	0.96485211	7.23	0.98712628
6.40	0.91924334	6.82	0.96562050	7.24	0.98745454
6.41	0.92073016	6.83	0.96637503	7.25	0.98777553
6.42	0.92219616	6.84	0.96711588	7.26	0.98808937
6.43	0.92364149	6.85	0.96784323	7.27	0.98839621
6.44	0.92506630	6.86	0.96855724	7.28	0.98869616
6.45	0.92647074	6.87	0.96925809	7.29	0.98898934

continued

Table A-8. (Continued) Probit Transformation

Probit	Proportion	Probit	Proportion	Probit	Proportion
7.30	0.98927589	7.73	0.99683328	8.16	0.99921115
7.31	0.98955592	7.74	0.99692804	8.17	0.99923781
7.32	0.98982956	7.75	0.99702024	8.18	0.99926362
7.33	0.99009692	7.76	0.99710993	8.19	0.99928864
7.34	0.99035813	7.77	0.99719719	8.20	0.99931286
7.35	0.99061329	7.78	0.99728206	8.21	0.99933633
7.36	0.99086253	7.79	0.99736460	8.22	0.99935905
7.37	0.99110596	7.80	0.99744487	8.23	0.99938105
7.38	0.99134368	7.81	0.99752293	8.24	0.99940235
7.39	0.99157581	7.82	0.99759882	8.25	0.99942297
7.40	0.99180246	7.83	0.99767260	8.26	0.99944294
7.41	0.99202374	7.84	0.99774432	8.27	0.99946226
7.42	0.99223975	7.85	0.99781404	8.28	0.99948096
7.43	0.99245059	7.86	0.99788179	8.29	0.99949906
7.44	0.99265637	7.87	0.99794764	8.30	0.99951658
7.45	0.99285719	7.88	0.99801162	8.31	0.99953352
7.46	0.99305315	7.89	0.99807379	8.32	0.99954991
7.47	0.99324435	7.90	0.99813419	8.33	0.99956577
7.48	0.99343088	7.91	0.99819286	8.34	0.99958111
7.49	0.99361285	7.92	0.99824984	8.35	0.99959594
7.50	0.99379033	7.93	0.99830519	8.36	0.99961029
7.51	0.99396344	7.94	0.99835894	8.37	0.99962416
7.52	0.99413226	7.95	0.99841113	8.38	0.99963757
7.53	0.99429687	7.96	0.99846180	8.39	0.99965054
7.54	0.99445738	7.97	0.99851100	8.40	0.99966307
7.55	0.99461385	7.98	0.99855876	8.41	0.99967519
7.56	0.99476639	7.99	0.99860511	8.42	0.99968689
7.57	0.99491507	8.00	0.99865010	8.43	0.99969821
7.58	0.99505998	8.01	0.99869376	8.44	0.99970914
7.59	0.99520120	8.02	0.99873613	8.45	0.99971971
7.60	0.99533881	8.03	0.99877723	8.46	0.99972991
7.61	0.99547289	8.04	0.99881711	8.47	0.99973977
7.62	0.95560351	8.05	0.99885579	8.48	0.99974929
7.63	0.99573076	8.06	0.99889332	8.49	0.99975849
7.64	0.99585470	8.07	0.99892971	8.50	0.99976737
7.65	0.99597541	8.08	0.99896500	8.51	0.99977595
7.66	0.99609297	8.09	0.99899922	8.52	0.99978423
7.67	0.99620744	8.10	0.99903240	8.53	0.99979222
7.68	0.99631889	8.11	0.99906456	8.54	0.99979994
7.69	0.99642740	8.12	0.99909574	8.55	0.99980738
7.70	0.99653303	8.13	0.99912597	8.56	0.99981457
7.71	0.99663584	8.14	0.99915526	8.57	0.99982151
7.72	0.99673590	8.15	0.99918365	8.58	0.99982820

Table A-8. (Continued) Probit Transformation

Probit	Proportion	Probit	Proportion	Probit	Proportion
8.59	0.99983466	8.73	0.99990426	8.87	0.99994558
8.60	0.99984089	8.74	0.99990799	8.88	0.99994777
8.61	0.99984690	8.75	0.99991158	8.89	0.99994988
8.62	0.99985270	8.76	0.99991504	8.90	0.99995190
8.63	0.99985829	8.77	0.99991838	8.91	0.99995385
8.64	0.99986368	8.78	0.99992159	8.92	0.99995573
8.65	0.99986888	8.79	0.99992468	8.93	0.99995753
8.66	0.99987389	8.80	0.99992765	8.94	0.99995926
8.67	0.99987872	8.81	0.99993052	8.95	0.99996092
8.68	0.99988338	8.82	0.99993327	8.96	0.99996253
8.69	0.99988787	8.83	0.99993593	8.97	0.99996406
8.70	0.99989220	8.84	0.99993848	8.98	0.99996554
8.71	0.99989637	8.85	0.99994094	8.99	0.99996696
8.72	0.99990039	8.86	0.99994331	9.00	0.99996833

Prepared from a program written by J.D. McCary.

Table A-9. Variance Ratio[a]

					$F(95\%)$[b]					
					n_1					
n_2	1	2	3	4	5	6	8	12	24	∞
1	161.4	199.5	215.7	224.6	230.2	234.0	238.9	243.9	249.0	254.3
2	18.51	19.00	19.16	19.25	19.30	19.33	19.37	19.41	19.45	19.50
3	10.13	9.55	9.28	9.12	9.01	8.94	8.84	8.74	8.64	8.53
4	7.71	6.94	6.59	6.39	6.26	6.16	6.04	5.91	5.77	5.63
5	6.61	5.79	5.41	5.19	5.05	4.95	4.82	4.68	4.53	4.36
6	5.99	5.14	4.76	4.53	4.39	4.28	4.15	4.00	3.84	3.67
7	5.59	4.74	4.35	4.12	3.97	3.87	3.73	3.57	3.41	3.23
8	5.32	4.46	4.07	3.84	3.69	3.58	3.44	3.28	3.12	2.93
9	5.12	4.26	3.86	3.63	3.48	3.37	3.23	3.07	2.90	2.71
10	4.96	4.10	3.71	3.48	3.33	3.22	3.07	2.91	2.74	2.54
11	4.84	3.98	3.59	3.36	3.20	3.09	2.95	2.79	2.61	2.40
12	4.75	3.88	3.49	3.26	3.11	3.00	2.85	2.69	2.50	2.30
13	4.67	3.80	3.41	3.18	3.02	2.92	2.77	2.60	2.42	2.21
14	4.60	3.74	3.34	3.11	2.96	2.85	2.70	2.53	2.35	2.13
15	4.54	3.68	3.29	3.06	2.90	2.79	2.64	2.48	2.29	2.07
16	4.49	3.63	3.24	3.01	2.85	2.74	2.59	2.42	2.24	2.01
17	4.45	3.59	3.20	2.96	2.81	2.70	2.55	2.38	2.19	1.96
18	4.41	3.55	3.16	2.93	2.77	2.66	2.51	2.34	2.15	1.92
19	4.38	3.52	3.13	2.90	2.74	2.63	2.48	2.31	2.11	1.88
20	4.35	3.49	3.10	2.87	2.71	2.60	2.45	2.28	2.08	1.84
21	4.32	3.47	3.07	2.84	2.68	2.57	2.42	2.25	2.05	1.81
22	4.30	3.44	3.05	2.82	2.66	2.55	2.40	2.23	2.03	1.78
23	4.28	3.42	3.03	2.80	2.64	2.53	2.38	2.20	2.00	1.76
24	4.26	3.40	3.01	2.78	2.62	2.51	2.36	2.18	1.98	1.73
25	4.24	3.38	2.99	2.76	2.60	2.49	2.34	2.16	1.96	1.71
26	4.22	3.37	2.98	2.74	2.59	2.47	2.32	2.15	1.95	1.69
27	4.21	3.35	2.96	2.73	2.57	2.46	2.30	2.13	1.93	1.67
28	4.20	3.34	2.95	2.71	2.56	2.44	2.29	2.12	1.91	1.65
29	4.18	3.33	2.93	2.70	2.54	2.43	2.28	2.10	1.90	1.64
30	4.17	3.32	2.92	2.69	2.53	2.42	2.27	2.09	1.89	1.62

Table A-9. (Continued) Variance Ratio[a]

					$F(95\%)$[b]					
					n_1					
n_2	1	2	3	4	5	6	8	12	24	∞
40	4.08	3.23	2.84	2.61	2.45	2.34	2.18	2.00	1.79	1.51
60	4.00	3.15	2.76	2.52	2.37	2.25	2.10	1.92	1.70	1.39
120	3.92	3.07	2.68	2.45	2.29	2.17	2.02	1.83	1.61	1.25
∞	3.84	2.99	2.60	2.37	2.21	2.10	1.94	1.75	1.52	1.00

[a] From Fisher, R. A. and Yates, F. (1963). Reprinted by permission of Addison Wesley Longman, Ltd. and Pearson Education, Ltd. Used with permission.

[b] Five percent points of F. Lower 5% points are found by interchange of $n1$ and n^2 — that is, n^1 must always correspond with the greater mean square, where n^1 and n^2 are appropriate degrees of freedom.

[c] One percent points of F. Lower % points are found by interchange of n^1 and n^2 — that is, n^1 must always correspond with the greater mean square, where n^1 and n^2 are appropriate degrees of freedom.

					$F(99\%)$[b]					
					n_1					
n_2	1	2	3	4	5	6	8	12	24	∞
1	4,052	4,999	5,403	5,625	5,764	5,859	5,982	6,106	6,234	6,366
2	98.50	99.00	99.17	99.25	99.30	99.33	99.37	99.42	99.46	99.50
3	34.12	30.82	29.46	28.71	28.24	27.91	27.49	27.05	26.60	26.12
4	21.20	18.00	16.69	15.98	15.52	15.21	14.80	14.37	13.93	13.46
5	16.26	13.27	12.06	11.39	10.97	10.67	10.29	9.89	9.47	9.02
6	13.74	10.92	9.78	9.15	8.75	8.47	8.10	7.72	7.31	6.88
7	12.25	9.55	8.45	7.85	7.46	7.19	6.84	6.47	6.07	5.65
8	11.26	8.65	7.59	7.01	6.63	6.37	6.03	5.67	5.28	4.86
9	10.56	8.02	6.99	6.42	6.06	5.80	5.47	5.11	4.73	4.31
10	10.04	7.56	6.55	5.99	5.64	5.39	5.06	4.71	4.33	3.91
11	9.65	7.20	6.22	5.67	5.32	5.07	4.74	4.40	4.02	3.60
12	9.33	6.93	5.95	5.41	5.06	4.82	4.50	4.16	3.78	3.36
13	9.07	6.70	5.74	5.20	4.86	4.62	4.30	3.96	3.59	3.16
14	8.86	6.51	5.56	5.03	4.69	4.46	4.14	3.80	3.43	3.00
15	8.68	6.36	5.42	4.89	4.56	4.32	4.00	3.67	3.29	2.87
16	8.53	6.23	5.29	4.77	4.44	4.20	3.89	3.55	3.18	2.75
17	8.40	6.11	5.18	4.67	4.34	4.10	3.79	3.45	3.08	2.65
18	8.28	6.01	5.09	4.58	4.25	4.01	3.71	3.37	3.00	2.57
19	8.18	5.93	5.01	4.50	4.17	3.94	3.63	3.30	2.92	2.49
20	8.10	5.85	4.94	4.43	4.10	3.87	3.56	3.23	2.86	2.42

continued

Table A-9. (Continued) Variance Ratio[a]

					$F(99\%)$[b]					
					n_1					
n_2	1	2	3	4	5	6	8	12	24	∞
21	8.02	5.78	4.87	4.37	4.04	3.81	3.51	3.17	2.80	2.36
22	7.94	5.72	4.82	4.31	3.99	3.76	3.45	3.12	2.75	2.31
23	7.88	5.66	4.76	4.26	3.94	3.71	3.41	3.07	2.70	2.26
24	7.82	5.61	4.72	4.22	3.90	3.67	3.36	3.03	2.66	2.21
25	7.77	5.57	4.68	4.18	3.86	3.63	3.32	2.99	2.62	2.17
26	7.72	5.53	4.64	4.14	3.82	3.59	3.29	2.96	2.58	2.13
27	7.68	5.49	4.60	4.11	3.78	3.56	3.26	2.93	2.55	2.10
28	7.64	5.45	4.57	4.07	3.75	3.53	3.23	2.90	2.52	2.06
29	7.60	5.42	4.54	4.04	3.73	3.50	3.20	2.87	2.49	2.03
30	7.56	5.39	4.51	4.02	3.70	3.47	3.17	2.84	2.47	2.01
40	7.31	5.18	4.31	3.83	3.51	3.29	2.99	2.66	2.29	1.80
60	7.08	4.98	4.13	3.65	3.34	3.12	2.82	2.50	2.12	1.60
120	6.85	4.79	3.95	3.48	3.17	2.96	2.66	2.34	1.95	1.38
∞	6.64	4.60	3.78	3.32	3.02	2.80	2.51	2.18	1.79	1.00

Table A-10. Critical Values of the q Distribution

				$\alpha = 0.05$					
v	$w = 2$	3	4	5	6	7	8	9	10
1	17.97	26.98	32.82	37.08	40.41	43.12	45.40	47.36	49.07
2	6.085	8.331	9.798	10.88	11.74	12.44	13.03	13.54	13.99
3	4.501	5.910	6.825	7.502	8.037	8.478	8.853	9.177	9.462
4	3.927	5.040	5.757	6.287	6.707	7.053	7.347	7.602	7.826
5	3.635	4.602	5.218	5.673	6.033	6.330	6.582	6.802	6.995
6	3.461	4.339	4.896	5.305	5.628	5.895	6.122	6.319	6.493
7	3.344	4.165	4.681	5.060	5.359	5.606	5.815	5.998	6.158
8	3.261	4.041	4.529	4.886	5.167	5.399	5.597	5.767	5.918
9	3.199	3.949	4.415	4.756	5.024	5.244	5.432	5.595	5.739
10	3.151	3.877	4.327	4.654	4.912	5.124	5.305	5.461	5.599
11	3.113	3.820	4.256	4.574	4.823	5.028	5.202	5.353	5,487
12	3.082	3.773	4.199	4.508	4.751	4.950	5.119	5.265	5.395
13	3.055	3.735	4.151	4.453	4.690	4.885	5.049	5.192	5.318
14	3.033	3.702	4.111	4.407	4.639	4.829	4.990	5.131	5.254
15	3.014	3.674	4.076	4.367	4.595	4.782	4.940	5.077	5.198
16	2.998	3.649	4.046	4.333	4.557	4.741	4.897	5.031	5.150
17	2.984	3.628	4.020	4.303	4.524	4.705	4.858	4.991	5.108
18	2.971	3.609	3.997	4.277	4.495	4.673	4.824	4.956	5.071
19	2.960	3.593	3.977	4.253	4.469	4.645	4.794	4.924	5.038
20	2.950	3.578	3.958	4.232	4.445	4.620	4.768	4.896	5.008
24	2.919	3.532	3.901	4.166	4.373	4.541	4.684	4.807	4.915
30	2.888	3.486	3.845	4.102	4.302	4.464	4.602	4.720	4.824
40	2.858	3.442	3.791	4.039	4.232	4.389	4.521	4.635	4.735
60	2.829	3.399	3.737	3.977	4.163	4.314	4.441	4.550	4.646
120	2.800	3.356	3.685	3.917	4.096	4.241	4.363	4.468	4.560
∞	2.772	3.314	3.633	3.858	4.030	4.170	4.286	4.387	3.474
v	$w = 11$	12	13	14	15	16	17	18	19
1	50.59	51.96	53.20	54.33	55.36	56.32	57.22	58.04	58.83
2	14.39	14.75	15.08	15.38	15.65	15.91	16.14	16.37	16.57
3	9.717	9.946	10.15	10.35	10.53	10.69	10.84	10.98	11.11
4	8.027	8.208	8.373	8.525	8.664	8.794	8.914	9.028	9.134
5	7.168	7.324	7.466	7.596	7.717	7.828	7.932	8.030	8.122
6	6.649	6.789	6.917	7.034	7.143	7.244	7.338	7.426	7.508
7	6.302	6.431	6.550	6.658	6.759	6.852	6.939	7.020	7.097
8	6.054	6.175	6.287	6.389	6.483	6.571	6.653	6.729	6.802

continued

Table A-10. (Continued) Critical Values of the q Distribution

v	$w = 11$	12	13	14	15	16	17	18	19
9	5.867	5.983	6.089	6.186	6.276	6.359	6.437	6.510	6.579
10	5.722	5.833	5.935	6.028	6.114	6.194	6.269	6.339	6.405
11	5.605	5.713	5.811	5.901	5.984	6.062	6.134	6.202	6.265
12	5.511	5.615	5.710	5.798	5.878	5.953	6.023	6.089	6.151
13	5.431	5.533	5.625	5.711	5.789	5.862	5.931	5.995	6.055
14	5.364	5.463	5.554	5.637	5.714	5.786	5.852	5.915	5.974
15	5.306	5.404	5.493	5.574	5.649	5.720	5.785	5.846	5.904
16	5.256	5.352	5.439	5.520	5.593	5.662	5.727	5.786	5.843
17	5.212	5.307	5.392	5.471	5.544	5.612	5.675	5.734	5.790
18	5.174	5.267	5.352	5.429	5.501	5.568	5.630	5.688	5.743
19	5.140	5.231	5.315	5.391	5.462	5.528	5.589	5.647	5.701
20	5.108	5.199	5.282	5.357	5.427	5.493	5.553	5.610	5.663
24	5.012	5.099	5.179	5.251	5.319	5.381	5.439	5.494	5.545
30	4.917	5.001	5.077	5.147	5.211	5.271	5.327	5.379	5.429
40	4.824	4.904	4.977	5.044	5.106	5.163	5.216	5.266	5.313
60	4.732	4.808	4.878	4.942	5.001	5.056	5.107	5.154	5.199
120	4.641	4.714	4.781	4.842	4.898	4.950	4.998	5.044	5.086
∞	4.552	4.622	4.685	4.743	4.796	4.845	4.891	4.934	4.974

$\alpha = 0.05$

v	$w = 20$	22	24	26	28	30	32	34	36
1	59.56	60.91	62.12	63.22	64.23	65.15	66.01	66.81	67.56
2	16.77	17.13	17.45	17.75	18.02	18.27	18.50	18.72	18.92
3	11.24	11.47	11.68	11.87	12.05	12.21	12.36	12.50	12.63
4	9.233	9.418	9.584	9.736	9.875	10.00	10.12	10.23	10.34
5	8.208	8.368	8.512	8.643	8.764	8.875	8.979	9.075	9.165
6	7.587	7.730	7.861	7.979	8.088	8.189	8.283	8.370	8.452
7	7.170	7.303	7.423	7.533	7.634	7.728	7.814	7.895	7.972
8	6.870	6.995	7.109	7.212	7.307	7.395	7.477	7.554	7.625
9	6.644	6.763	6.871	6.970	7.061	7.145	7.222	7.295	7.363
10	6.467	6.582	6.686	6.781	6.868	6.948	7.023	7.093	7.159
11	6.326	6.436	6.536	6.628	6.712	6.790	6.863	6.930	6.994
12	6.209	6.317	6.414	6.503	6.585	6.600	6.731	6.796	6.858
13	6.112	6.217	6.312	6.398	6.478	6.551	6.620	6.684	6.744
14	6.029	6.132	6.224	6.309	6.387	6.459	6.526	6.588	6.647
15	5.958	6.059	6.149	6.233	6.309	6.379	6.445	6.506	6.564

Table A-10. (Continued) Critical Values of the q Distribution

				$\alpha = 0.05$					
v	$w = 20$	22	24	26	28	30	32	34	36
16	5.897	5.995	6.084	6.166	6.241	6.310	6.374	6.434	6.491
17	5.842	5.940	6.027	6.107	6.181	6.249	6.313	6.372	6.427
18	5.794	5.890	5.977	6.055	6.128	6.195	6.258	6.316	6.371
19	5.752	5.846	5.932	6.009	6.081	6.147	6.209	6.267	6.321
20	5.714	5.807	5.891	5.968	6.039	6.104	6.165	6.222	6.275
24	5.594	5.683	5.764	5.838	5.906	5.968	6.027	6.081	6.132
30	5.475	5.561	5.638	5.709	5.774	5.833	5.889	5.941	5.990
40	5.358	5.439	5.513	5.581	5.642	5.700	5.753	5.803	5.849
60	5.241	5.319	5.389	5.453	5.512	5.566	5.617	5.664	5.708
120	5.126	5.200	5.266	5.327	5.382	5.434	5.481	5.526	5.568
∞	5.012	5.081	5.144	5.201	5.253	5.301	5.346	5.388	5.427

v	$w = 38$	40	50	60	70	80	90	100	
1	68.26	68.92	71.73	73.97	75.82	77.40	78.77	78.98	
2	19.11	19.28	20.05	20.66	21.16	21.59	21.96	22.29	
3	12.75	12.87	13.36	13.76	14.08	14.36	14.61	14.82	
4	10.44	10.53	10.93	11.24	11.51	11.73	11.92	12.09	
5	9.250	9.330	9.674	9.949	10.18	10.38	10.54	10.69	
6	8.529	8.601	8.913	9.163	9.370	9.548	9.702	9.839	
7	8.043	8.110	8.400	8.632	8.824	8.989	9.133	9.261	
8	7.693	7.756	8.029	8.248	8.430	8.586	8.722	8.843	
9	7.428	7.488	7.749	7.958	8.132	8.281	8.410	8.526	
10	7.220	7.279	7.529	7.730	7.897	8.041	8.166	8.276	
11	7.053	7.110	7.352	7.546	7.708	7.847	7.968	8.075	
12	6.916	6.970	7.205	7.394	7.552	7.687	7.804	7.909	
13	6.800	6.854	7.083	7.267	7.421	7.552	7.667	7.769	
14	6.702	6.754	6.979	7.159	7.309	7.438	7.550	7.650	
15	6.618	6.669	6.888	7.065	7.212	7.339	7.449	7.546	
16	6.544	6.594	6.810	6.984	7.128	7.252	7.360	7.457	
17	6.479	6.529	6.741	6.912	7.054	7.176	7.283	7.377	
18	6.422	6.471	6.680	6.848	6.989	7.100	7.218	7.307	
19	6.371	6.419	6.626	6.792	6.930	7.048	7.152	7.244	
20	6.325	6.373	6.576	6.740	6.877	6.994	7.097	7.187	

continued

Table A-10. (Continued) Critical Values of the q Distribution

v	$w = 38$	40	50	60	70	80	90	100
24	6.181	6.226	6.421	6.579	6.710	6.822	6.920	7.008
30	6.037	6.080	6.267	6.417	6.543	6.650	6.744	6.827
40	5.893	5.934	6.112	6.255	6.375	6.477	6.566	6.645
60	5.750	5.789	5.958	6.093	6.206	6.303	6.387	6.462
120	5.607	5.644	5.802	5.929	6.035	6.126	6.205	6.275
∞	5.463	5.498	5.646	5.764	5.863	5.947	6.020	6.085

<table>
<tr><td colspan="10" align="center">$\alpha = 0.01$</td></tr>
<tr><td>v</td><td>$w = 2$</td><td>3</td><td>4</td><td>5</td><td>6</td><td>7</td><td>8</td><td>9</td><td>10</td></tr>
<tr><td>1</td><td>90.03</td><td>135.0</td><td>164.3</td><td>185.6</td><td>202.2</td><td>215.8</td><td>227.2</td><td>237.0</td><td>245.6</td></tr>
<tr><td>2</td><td>14.04</td><td>19.02</td><td>22.29</td><td>24.72</td><td>26.63</td><td>28.20</td><td>29.53</td><td>30.68</td><td>31.69</td></tr>
<tr><td>3</td><td>8.261</td><td>10.62</td><td>12.17</td><td>13.33</td><td>14.24</td><td>15.00</td><td>15.64</td><td>16.20</td><td>16.69</td></tr>
<tr><td>4</td><td>6.512</td><td>8.120</td><td>9.173</td><td>9.958</td><td>10.58</td><td>11.10</td><td>11.55</td><td>11.93</td><td>12.27</td></tr>
<tr><td>5</td><td>5.702</td><td>6.976</td><td>7.804</td><td>8.421</td><td>8.913</td><td>9.321</td><td>9.669</td><td>9.972</td><td>10.24</td></tr>
<tr><td>6</td><td>5.243</td><td>6.331</td><td>7.033</td><td>7.556</td><td>7.973</td><td>8.318</td><td>8.613</td><td>8.869</td><td>9.097</td></tr>
<tr><td>7</td><td>4.949</td><td>5.919</td><td>6.543</td><td>7.005</td><td>7.373</td><td>7.679</td><td>7.939</td><td>8.166</td><td>8.368</td></tr>
<tr><td>8</td><td>4.746</td><td>5.635</td><td>6.204</td><td>6.625</td><td>6.960</td><td>7.237</td><td>7.474</td><td>7,681</td><td>7.863</td></tr>
<tr><td>9</td><td>4.596</td><td>5.428</td><td>5.957</td><td>6.348</td><td>6.658</td><td>6.915</td><td>7.134</td><td>7.325</td><td>7.495</td></tr>
<tr><td>10</td><td>4.482</td><td>5.270</td><td>5.769</td><td>6.136</td><td>6.428</td><td>6.669</td><td>6.875</td><td>7.055</td><td>7.213</td></tr>
<tr><td>11</td><td>4.392</td><td>5.146</td><td>5.621</td><td>5.970</td><td>6.247</td><td>6.476</td><td>6.672</td><td>6.842</td><td>6.992</td></tr>
<tr><td>12</td><td>4.320</td><td>5.046</td><td>5.502</td><td>5.836</td><td>6.101</td><td>6.321</td><td>6.507</td><td>6.670</td><td>6.814</td></tr>
<tr><td>13</td><td>4.260</td><td>4.964</td><td>5.404</td><td>5.727</td><td>5.981</td><td>6.192</td><td>6.372</td><td>6.528</td><td>6.667</td></tr>
<tr><td>14</td><td>4.210</td><td>4.895</td><td>5.322</td><td>5.634</td><td>5.881</td><td>6.085</td><td>6.258</td><td>6.409</td><td>6.543</td></tr>
<tr><td>15</td><td>4.168</td><td>4.836</td><td>5.252</td><td>5.556</td><td>5.796</td><td>5.994</td><td>6.162</td><td>6.309</td><td>6.439</td></tr>
<tr><td>16</td><td>4.131</td><td>4.786</td><td>5.192</td><td>5.489</td><td>5.722</td><td>5.915</td><td>6.079</td><td>6.222</td><td>6.349</td></tr>
<tr><td>17</td><td>4.099</td><td>4.742</td><td>5.140</td><td>5.430</td><td>5.659</td><td>5.847</td><td>6.007</td><td>6.147</td><td>6.270</td></tr>
<tr><td>18</td><td>4.071</td><td>4.703</td><td>5.094</td><td>5.379</td><td>5.603</td><td>5.788</td><td>5.944</td><td>6.081</td><td>6.201</td></tr>
<tr><td>19</td><td>4.046</td><td>4.670</td><td>5.054</td><td>5.334</td><td>5.554</td><td>5.735</td><td>5.889</td><td>6.022</td><td>6.141</td></tr>
<tr><td>20</td><td>4.024</td><td>4.639</td><td>5.018</td><td>5.294</td><td>5.510</td><td>5.688</td><td>5.839</td><td>5.970</td><td>6.087</td></tr>
<tr><td>24</td><td>3.956</td><td>4.546</td><td>4.907</td><td>5.168</td><td>5.374</td><td>5.542</td><td>5.685</td><td>5.809</td><td>5.919</td></tr>
<tr><td>30</td><td>3.889</td><td>4.455</td><td>4.799</td><td>5.048</td><td>5.242</td><td>5.401</td><td>5.536</td><td>5.653</td><td>5.756</td></tr>
<tr><td>40</td><td>3.825</td><td>4.367</td><td>4.696</td><td>4.931</td><td>5.114</td><td>5.265</td><td>5.392</td><td>5.502</td><td>5.559</td></tr>
<tr><td>60</td><td>3.762</td><td>4.282</td><td>4.595</td><td>4,818</td><td>4.991</td><td>5.133</td><td>5.253</td><td>5.356</td><td>5.447</td></tr>
<tr><td>120</td><td>3.702</td><td>4.200</td><td>4.497</td><td>4.709</td><td>4.872</td><td>5.005</td><td>5.118</td><td>5.214</td><td>5.299</td></tr>
<tr><td>∞</td><td>3.643</td><td>4.120</td><td>4.403</td><td>4.603</td><td>4.757</td><td>4.882</td><td>4.987</td><td>5.078</td><td>5.157</td></tr>
</table>

Table A-10. (Continued) Critical Values of the q Distribution

v	$w = 11$	12	13	14	15	16	17	18	19
1	253.2	260.0	266.2	271.8	277.0	281.8	286.3	290.4	294.3
2	32.59	33.40	34.13	34.81	35.43	36.00	36.53	37.03	37.50
3	17.13	17.53	17.89	18.22	18.52	18.81	19.07	19.32	19.55
4	12.57	12.84	13.09	13.32	13.53	13.73	13.91	14.08	14.24
5	10.48	10.70	10.89	11.08	11.24	11.40	11.55	11.68	11.81
6	9.301	9.485	9.653	9.808	9.951	10.08	10.21	10.32	10.43
7	8.548	8.711	8.860	8.997	9.124	9.242	9.353	9.456	9.554
8	8.027	8.176	8.312	8.436	8.552	8.659	8.760	8.854	8.943
9	7.647	7.784	7.910	8.025	8.132	8.232	8.325	8.412	8.495
10	7.356	7.485	7.603	7.712	7.812	7.906	7.993	8.076	8.153
11	7.128	7.250	7.362	7.465	7.560	7.649	7.732	7.809	7.883
12	6.943	7.060	7.167	7.265	7.356	7.441	7.520	7.594	7.665
13	6.791	6.903	7.006	7.101	7.188	7.269	7.345	7.417	7.485
14	6.664	6.772	6.871	6.962	7.047	7.126	7.199	7.268	7.333
15	6.555	6.660	6.757	6.845	6.927	7.003	7.074	7.142	7.204
16	6.462	6.564	6.658	6.744	6.823	6.898	6.967	7.032	7.093
17	6.381	6.480	6.572	6.656	6.734	6.806	6.873	6.937	6.997
18	6.310	6.407	6.497	6.579	6.655	6.725	6.792	6.854	6.912
19	6.247	6.342	6.430	6.510	6.585	6.654	6.719	6.780	6.837
20	6.191	6.285	6.371	6.450	6.523	6.591	6.654	6.714	6.771
24	6.017	6.106	6.186	6.261	6.330	6.394	6.453	6.510	6.563
30	5.849	5.932	6.008	6.078	6.143	6.203	6.259	6.311	6.361
40	5.686	5.764	5.835	5.900	5.961	6.017	6.069	6.119	6.165
60	5.528	5.601	5.667	5.728	5.785	5.837	5.886	5.931	5.974
120	5.375	5.443	5.505	5.562	5.614	5.662	5.708	5.750	5.790
∞	5.227	5.290	5.348	5.400	5.448	5.493	5.535	5.574	5.611

$\alpha = 0.01$

v	$w = 20$	22	24	26	28	30	32	34	36
1	298.0	304.7	310.8	316.3	321.3	326.0	330.3	334.3	338.0
2	37.95	38.76	39.49	40.15	40.76	41.32	41.84	42.33	42.78
3	19.77	20.17	20.53	20.86	21.16	21.44	21.70	21.95	22.17
4	14.40	14.68	14.93	15.16	15.37	15.57	15.75	15.92	16.08
5	11.93	12.16	12.36	12.54	12.71	12.87	13.02	13.15	13.28

continued

Table A-10. (Continued) Critical Values of the q Distribution

v	$w = 20$	22	24	26	28	30	32	34	36
6	10.54	10.73	10.91	11.06	11.21	11.34	11.47	11.58	11.69
7	9.646	9.815	9.970	10.11	10.24	10.36	10.47	10.58	10.67
8	9.027	9.182	9.322	9.450	9.569	9.678	9.779	9.874	9.964
9	8.573	8.717	8.847	8.966	9.075	9.177	9.271	9.360	9.443
10	8.226	8.361	8.483	8.595	8.698	8.794	8.883	8.966	9.044
11	7.952	8.080	8.196	8.303	8.400	8.491	8.575	8.654	8.728
12	7.731	7.853	7.964	8.066	8.159	8.246	8.327	8.402	8.473
13	7.548	7.665	7.772	7.870	7.960	8.043	8.121	8.193	8.262
14	7.395	7.508	7.611	7.705	7.792	7.873	7.948	8.018	8.084
15	7.264	7.374	7.474	7.566	7.650	7.728	7.800	7.869	7.932
16	7.152	7.258	7.356	7.445	7.527	7.602	7.673	7.339	7.802
17	7.053	7.158	7.253	7.340	7.420	7.493	7.563	7.627	7.687
18	6.968	7.070	7.163	7.247	7.325	7.398	7.465	7.528	7.587
19	6.891	6.992	7.082	7.166	7.242	7.313	7.379	7.440	7.498
20	6.823	6.922	7.011	7.092	7.168	7.237	7.302	7.362	7.419
24	6.612	6.705	6.789	6.865	6.936	7.001	7.062	7.119	7.173
30	6.407	6.494	6.572	6.644	6.710	6.772	6.828	6.881	6.932
40	6.209	6.289	6.362	6.429	6.490	6.547	6.600	6.650	6.697
60	6.015	6.090	6.158	6.220	6.277	6.330	6.378	6.424	6.467
120	5.827	5.897	5.959	6.016	6.069	6.117	6.162	6.204	6.244
∞	5.645	5.709	5.766	5.818	5.866	5.911	5.952	5.990	6.026

v	$w = 38$	40	50	60	70	80	90	100
1	341.5	344.8	358.9	370.1	379.4	387.3	394.1	400.1
2	43.21	43.61	45.53	46.70	47.83	48.80	49.64	50.38
3	22.39	22.59	23.45	24.13	24.71	25.19	25.62	25.99
4	16.23	16.37	16.98	17.46	17.86	18.02	18.50	18.77
5	13.40	13.52	14.00	14.39	14.72	14.99	15.23	15.45
6	11.80	11.90	12.31	12.65	12.92	13.16	13.37	13.55
7	10.77	10.85	11.23	11.52	11.77	11.99	12.17	12.34
8	10.05	10.13	10.47	10.75	10.97	11.17	11.34	11.49
9	9.521	9.594	9.912	10.17	10.38	10.57	10.73	10.87
10	9.117	9.187	9.486	9.726	9.927	10.10	10.25	10.39

Table A-10. (Continued) Critical Values of the q Distribution

v	$w = 38$	40	50	60	70	80	90	100
11	8.798	8.864	9.148	9.377	9.568	9.732	9.875	10.00
12	8.539	8.603	8.875	9.094	9.277	9.434	9.571	9.693
13	8.326	8.387	8.648	8.859	9.035	9.187	9.318	9.436
14	8.146	8.204	8.457	8.661	8.832	8.978	9.106	9.219
15	7.992	8.049	8.295	8.492	8.658	8.800	8.924	9.035
16	7.860	7.916	8.154	8.347	8.507	8.646	8.767	8.874
17	7.745	7.799	8.031	8.219	8.377	8.511	8.630	8.735
18	7.643	7.696	7.924	8.107	8.261	8.393	8.508	8.611
19	7.553	7.605	7.828	8.008	8.159	8.288	8.401	8.502
20	7.473	7.523	7.742	7.919	8.067	8.194	8.305	8.404
24	7.223	7.270	7.476	7.642	7.780	7.900	8.004	8.097
30	6.978	7.023	7.215	7.370	7.500	7.611	7.709	7.796
40	6.740	6.782	6.960	7.104	7.225	7.328	7.419	7.500
60	6.507	6.546	6.710	6.843	6.954	7.050	7.133	7.207
120	6.281	6.316	6.467	6.588	6.689	6.776	6.852	6.919
∞	6.060	6.092	6.228	6.338	6.429	6.507	6.575	6.636

Reprinted from Tallarida, R.J. and Murray, R.B., *Manual of Pharmacologic Calculations with Computer Programs*, 2nd ed 1987. By permission of Springer-Verlag, New York.

Table A-11A. Probabilities Associated with Values as Small as Observed Values of U in the Mann-Whitney Test

$[n_2 = 3]$

	n_1		
U	1	2	3
0	0.250	0.100	0.050
1	0.500	0.200	0.100
2	0.750	0.400	0.200
3		0.600	0.350
4			0.500
5			0.650

$[n_2 = 4]$

	n_1			
U	1	2	3	4
0	0.200	0.067	0.028	0.014
1	0.400	0.133	0.057	0.029
2	0.600	0.267	0.114	0.057
3		0.400	0.200	0.100
4		0.600	0.314	0.171
5			0.429	0.243
6			0.571	0.343
7				0.443
8				0.557

$[n_2 = 5]$

	n_1				
U	1	2	3	4	5
0	0.167	0.047	0.018	0.008	0.004
1	0.333	0.095	0.036	0.016	0.008
2	0.500	0.190	0.071	0.032	0.016
3	0.067	0.286	0.125	0.056	0.028
4		0.429	0.196	0.095	0.048
5		0.571	0.286	0.143	0.075
6			0.393	0.206	0.111
7			0.500	0.278	0.155
8			0.607	0.365	0.210
9				0.452	0.274

$[n_2 = 6]$

	n_1					
U	1	2	3	4	5	6
0	0.143	0.036	0.012	0.005	0.002	0.001
1	0.286	0.071	0.024	0.010	0.004	0.002
2	0.428	0.143	0.048	0.019	0.009	0.004
3	0.571	0.214	0.083	0.033	0.015	0.008
4		0.321	0.131	0.057	0.026	0.013
5		0.429	0.190	0.086	0.041	0.021
6		0.571	0.274	0.129	0.063	0.032
7			0.357	0.176	0.089	0.047
8			0.452	0.238	0.123	0.066
9			0.548	0.305	0.165	0.090

$[n_2 = 5]$

n_1

U	1	2	3	4	5
10				0.548	0.345
11					0.421
12					0.500
13					0.579

$[n_2 = 6]$

n_1

U	1	2	3	4	5	6
10				0.381	0.214	0.120
11				0.457	0.268	0.155
12				0.545	0.331	0.197
13					0.396	0.242
14					0.465	0.294
15					0.535	0.350
16						0.409
17						0.469
18						0.531

continued

Table A-11A. (Continued) Probabilities Associated with Values as Small as Observed Values of U in the Mann-Whitney Test[a]

$[n_2 = 7]$

U	n_1						
	1	2	3	4	5	6	7
0	0.125	0.028	0.008	0.003	0.001	0.001	0.000
1	0.250	0.056	0.017	0.006	0.003	0.001	0.001
2	0.375	0.111	0.033	0.012	0.005	0.002	0.001
3	0.500	0.167	0.058	0.021	0.009	0.004	0.002
4	0.625	0.250	0.092	0.036	0.015	0.007	0.003
5		0.333	0.133	0.055	0.024	0.011	0.006
6		0.444	0.192	0.082	0.037	0.017	0.009
7		0.556	0.258	0.115	0.053	0.026	0.013
8			0.333	0.158	0.074	0.037	0.019
9			0.417	0.206	0.101	0.051	0.027
10			0.500	0.264	0.134	0.069	0.036
11			0.583	0.324	0.172	0.090	0.049
12				0.394	0.216	0.117	0.064
13				0.464	0.265	0.147	0.082
14				0.538	0.319	0.183	0.104
15					0.378	0.223	0.130
16					0.438	0.267	0.159
17					0.500	0.314	0.191
18					0.562	0.365	0.228
19						0.418	0.267
20						0.473	0.310
21						0.527	0.355
22							0.402
23							0.451
24							0.500
25							0.549

$[n_2 = 8]$

U	n_1								t	Normal
	1	2	3	4	5	6	7	8		
0	0.111	0.022	0.006	0.002	0.001	0.000	0.000	0.000	3.308	0.001
1	0.222	0.044	0.012	0.004	0.002	0.001	0.000	0.000	3.203	0.001
2	0.333	0.089	0.024	0.008	0.003	0.001	0.001	0.000	3.098	0.001
3	0.444	0.133	0.042	0.014	0.005	0.002	0.001	0.001	3.993	0.001
4	0.556	0.200	0.067	0.024	0.009	0.004	0.002	0.001	3.888	0.002
5		0.267	0.097	0.036	0.015	0.006	0.003	0.001	2.783	0.003
6		0.356	0.139	0.055	0.023	0.010	0.005	0.002	2.678	0.004
7		0.444	0.188	0.077	0.033	0.015	0.007	0.003	2.573	0.005
8		0.556	0.248	0.107	0.047	0.021	0.010	0.005	2.468	0.007
9			0.315	0.141	0.064	0.030	0.014	0.007	2.363	0.009
10			0.387	0.184	0.085	0.041	0.020	0.010	2.258	0.012
11			0.461	0.230	0.111	0.054	0.027	0.014	2.153	0.016
12			0.539	0.285	0.142	0.071	0.036	0.019	2.048	0.020
13				0.341	0.177	0.091	0.047	0.025	1.943	0.026
14				0.404	0.217	0.114	0.060	0.032	1.838	0.033
15				0.467	0.262	0.141	0.076	0.041	1.733	0.041
16				0.533	0.311	0.172	0.095	0.052	1.628	0.052
17					0.362	0.207	0.116	0.065	1.523	0.064
18					0.416	0.245	0.140	0.080	1.418	0.078

continued

Table A-11A. (Continued) Probabilities Associated with Values as Small as Observed Values of U in the Mann-Whitney Test[a]

$[n_2 = 8]$

U	1	2	3	4	5	6	7	8	t	Normal
19					0.472	0.286	0.168	0.097	1.313	0.094
20					0.528	0.331	0.198	0.117	1.208	0.113
21						0.377	0.232	0.139	1.102	0.135
22						0.426	0.268	0.164	0.998	0.159
23						0.475	0.306	0.191	0.893	0.185
24						0.525	0.347	0.221	0.788	0.215
25							0.389	0.253	0.683	0.247
26							0.433	0.287	0.578	0.282
27							0.478	0.323	0.473	0.318
28							0.522	0.360	0.368	0.356
29								0.399	0.263	0.396
30								0.439	0.158	0.437
31								0.480	0.052	0.481
32								0.520		

Table A-11B. Critical Values of U in the Mann-Whitney Test: Critical Values of U for a One-Tailed Test at $\alpha = 0.001$ or for a Two-Tailed Test at $\alpha = 0.002$

n_1	9	10	11	12	13	14	15	16	17	18	19	20
1												
2												
3									0	0	0	0
4		0	0	0	1	1	1	2	2	3	3	3
5	1	1	2	2	3	3	4	5	5	6	7	7
6	2	3	4	4	5	6	7	8	9	10	11	12
7	3	5	6	7	8	9	10	11	13	14	15	16
8	5	6	8	9	11	12	14	15	17	18	20	21
9	7	8	10	12	14	15	17	19	21	23	25	26
10	8	10	12	14	17	19	21	23	25	27	29	32
11	10	12	15	17	20	22	24	27	29	32	34	37
12	12	14	17	20	23	25	28	31	34	37	40	42
13	14	17	20	23	26	29	32	35	38	42	45	48
14	15	19	22	25	29	32	36	39	43	46	50	54
15	17	21	24	28	32	36	40	43	47	51	55	59
16	19	23	27	31	35	39	43	48	52	56	60	65
17	21	25	29	34	38	43	47	52	57	61	66	70
18	23	27	32	37	42	46	51	56	61	66	71	76
19	25	29	34	40	45	50	55	60	66	71	77	82
20	26	32	37	42	48	54	59	65	70	76	82	88

Critical Values of U for a One-Tailed Test at $\alpha = 0.01$ or for a Two-Tailed Test at $\alpha = 0.02$

n_1	9	10	11	12	13	14	15	16	17	18	19	20
1												
2					0	0	0	0	0	0	1	1
3	1	1	1	2	2	2	3	3	4	4	4	5
4	3	3	4	5	5	6	7	7	8	9	9	10
5	5	6	7	8	9	10	11	12	13	14	15	16
6	7	8	9	11	12	13	15	16	18	19	20	22
7	9	11	12	14	16	17	19	21	23	24	26	28
8	11	13	15	17	20	22	24	26	28	30	32	34
9	14	16	18	21	23	26	28	31	33	36	38	40
10	16	19	22	24	27	30	33	36	38	41	44	47
11	18	22	25	28	31	34	37	41	44	47	50	53
12	21	24	28	31	35	38	42	46	49	53	56	60

continued

Table A-11B. (Continued) Critical Values of U for a One-Tailed Test at $\alpha =$ 0.01 or for a Two-Tailed Test at $\alpha = 0.02$

n_1						$[n_2]$						
	9	10	11	12	13	14	15	16	17	18	19	20
13	23	27	31	35	39	43	47	51	55	59	63	67
14	26	30	34	38	43	47	51	56	60	65	69	73
15	28	33	37	42	47	51	56	61	66	70	75	80
16	31	36	41	46	51	56	61	66	71	76	82	87
17	33	38	44	49	55	60	66	71	77	82	88	93
18	36	41	47	53	59	65	70	76	82	88	94	100
19	38	44	50	56	63	69	75	82	88	94	101	107
20	40	47	53	60	67	73	80	87	93	100	107	114

Critical Values of U for a One-Tailed Test at $\alpha = 0.025$ or for a Two-Tailed Test at $\alpha = 0.05$

	9	10	11	12	13	14	15	16	17	18	19	20
1												
2	0	0	0	1	1	1	1	1	2	2	2	2
3	2	3	3	4	4	5	5	6	6	7	7	8
4	4	5	6	7	8	9	10	11	11	12	13	13
5	7	8	9	11	12	13	14	15	17	18	19	20
6	10	11	13	14	16	17	19	21	22	24	25	27
7	12	14	16	18	20	22	24	26	28	30	32	34
8	15	17	19	22	24	26	29	31	34	36	38	41
9	17	20	23	26	28	31	34	37	39	42	45	48
10	20	23	26	29	33	36	39	42	45	48	52	55
11	23	26	30	33	37	40	44	47	51	55	58	62
12	26	29	33	37	41	45	49	53	57	61	65	69
13	28	33	37	41	45	50	54	59	63	67	72	76
14	31	36	40	45	50	55	59	64	67	74	78	83
15	34	39	44	49	54	59	64	70	75	80	85	90
16	37	42	47	53	59	64	70	75	81	86	92	98
17	39	45	51	57	63	67	75	81	87	93	99	105
18	42	48	55	61	67	74	80	86	93	99	106	112
19	45	52	58	65	72	78	85	92	99	106	113	119
20	48	55	62	69	76	83	90	98	105	112	119	127

Critical Values of U for a One-Tailed Test at $\alpha = 0.05$ or for a Two-Tailed Test at $\alpha = 0.10$

n_2						$[n_1]$						
	9	10	11	12	13	14	15	16	17	18	19	20
1											0	0
2	1	1	1	2	2	2	3	3	3	4	4	4
3	3	4	5	5	6	7	7	8	9	9	10	11
4	6	7	8	9	10	11	12	14	15	16	17	18
5	9	11	12	13	15	16	18	19	20	22	23	25

Table A-11B. (Continued) Critical Values of U for a One-Tailed Test at α = 0.05 or for a Two-Tailed Test at α = 0.10

						$[n_1]$						
n_2	9	10	11	12	13	14	15	16	17	18	19	20
6	12	14	16	17	19	21	23	25	26	28	30	32
7	15	17	19	21	24	26	28	30	33	35	37	39
8	18	20	23	26	28	31	33	36	39	41	44	47
9	21	24	27	30	33	36	39	42	45	48	51	54
10	24	27	31	34	37	41	44	48	51	55	58	62
11	27	31	34	38	42	46	50	54	57	61	65	69
12	30	34	38	42	47	51	55	60	64	68	72	77
13	33	37	42	47	51	56	61	65	70	75	80	84
14	36	41	46	51	56	61	66	71	77	82	87	92
15	39	44	50	55	61	66	72	77	83	88	94	100
16	42	48	54	60	65	71	77	83	89	95	101	107
17	45	51	57	64	70	77	83	89	96	102	109	115
18	48	55	61	68	75	82	88	95	102	109	116	123
19	51	58	65	72	80	87	94	101	109	116	123	130
20	54	62	69	77	84	92	100	107	115	123	130	138

Index